# LOVE FOOD

# THAT LOVES YOU BACK

## LIFE FULLY NOURISHED IS DELICIOUS

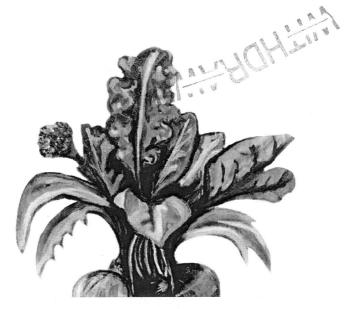

Presented to

**Spring Branch Memorial Library**

By

**Friends of the Library with Buy
A Book Campaign Funds**

Harris County
Public Library
*your pathway to knowledge*

## DOROTHY HOLTERMANN

Contact Dorothy Holtermann at www.nurturenaturenutrition.com

Prepublication technical assistance and editing by LOTONtech Limited (www.lotontech.com).

Print ISBN-13: 978-0692426821

Print ISBN-10: 0692426825

Published by Artbinders LLC

Contact the publisher at www.artbinders.com

Come visit my website at www.nurturenaturenutrition.com for free offers or to contact me. I am offering new delicious recipes and nutrition tips. I am also offering private and group nutrition and nourishment counseling, plus original and fantastic retreat and class opportunities. See you there!

Or contact me at coachdorothyholtermann@gmail.com.

Because life fully nourished is delicious…

# Contents

## Praise for the Author and the Book

*"In my first year of knowing Dorothy, she completely transformed physically, emotionally, and spiritually, in a way that is truly miraculous. With her beautiful, courageous heart, Dorothy is a force in the evolution, growth, and healing of herself and of others."*

Dr. Adam Turner, MD

*"If you are looking for a knowledgeable, compassionate, and insightful guide on your healing journey, Dorothy Holtermann is a natural healer with whom you should consider working. Dorothy possesses that rare combination of talents—deep knowledge of the healing arts, warm-hearted openness with her clients, and the ability to work with the whole human being, employing a wide array of modalities to bring about the restoration of body, mind, heart, and soul."*

Tom Monte
Bestselling Author and Counselor

*"I have known Dorothy both professionally & personally for quite some time, and observing her transformation has been awe-inspiring. She is a brilliant seeker, whose incredible heart & extensive nutritional knowledge will no doubt contribute significantly to the quantum shift in enhancing the longevity of our species. We are truly blessed for this Agent of Change at such a critical juncture in our history."*

Dr. Cliff Inkles, DC

*"Love Food That Loves You Back is a book that will provide you with a foundation of conscious and healthy eating. All too often we eat out of emotional, rather than physical need. Dorothy is a true testimony in how her knowledge of healthy eating empowered her to heal herself through whole foods."*

Margaret Torrellas
Professor of Psychology

*"Dorothy took the skill of organizing to a new level of greatness. As a participant in the TM training that she coordinated, I was beyond impressed with her clarity and consideration. She went above and beyond to accommodate my limitations with grace and understanding."*

Cody Schreger
CHHC

*"I had just turned 40, I was tired & stressed out. I have worked as a nurse for the past 20 years helping people daily, but I was having trouble helping myself. I was in a funk! Dorothy was amazing! Through her guidance, I made some subtle changes in my diet, I began to meditate along with my yoga practice. Dorothy coached me into a better state of wellness & I now feel better than I ever have!"*

Dawn Nowak
Nurse

*"Dorothy is a powerful intuitive healer. She has personally provided me with effective nutritional counseling that has shifted the way I look at food as well as how I view myself. I realized through her guidance that my relationship with food had a lot to do with beliefs about myself. She has led me to a clearer understanding of self and has given me tools to eat for my body and my health."*

Larissa Schiano
Founder of Living Through Motion and Yoga Teacher

*"Dorothy is an inspirational leader. She offers us her vast knowledge of nutrition and natural healing with passion and kindness. Her philosophy to "love food that loves you back" leads us to discover a new world of food that nourishes and heals our body and our life."* I have attended two of her workshops and they have changed the way I think about food forever.

Chisako Liu
Fashion Executive

*"Dorothy Holtermann is an exceptionally thoughtful and caring person. Her generous spirit was appreciated not only by me but by everyone participating in the successful TM and Ayurveda workshops I taught in NYC that she had organized."*

Prudence Farrow Bruns, PhD, subject of Beatles Song "Dear Prudence"

*"I have recently had the privilege of being a part of Dorothy's group health sessions. What I learned in 4 sessions far surpassed what I have read in dozens of health books. I was served tea, spoken to with love, and shared health failures and success with the entire group. She gave us individual direction for an improved healthy life plus overall discussions in the area of inflammation, cooking techniques, shopping tips, and so much more. Thank you Dorothy for all your guidance. I will implement all of what you taught me."*

Rita Grudzinski
Yoga Teacher, Age 47

*"The encouragement, support, and just the plain good sound advice I received from Dorothy Holtermann as I pursued a new career direction assisted me greatly on my path. When there was confusion, worry, doubt or stress seemingly in the way, and no matter how hectic life was, Dorothy helped me to fuel my dream to fruition. Change, even for the better, can be difficult. I am so glad I didn't even think twice about reaching out for her assistance through my career transition. Dorothy has the rare gift to embolden one with confidence and practical problem solving which eases all the other interfering factors that can present themselves when there is change. With her coaching I was able to maintain my equilibrium throughout, along with the perfectly composed professional demeanor I desired. Thank you Dorothy!"*

Ruth Davidson Hahn
Dance for Parkinson's Program Director, Age 58

*"Dorothy Holtermann is a never ending source of health and wellness information. She is also a beautiful, compassionate person who is very easy to talk to. Between*

*Dorothy's health coaching and my yoga practice, at 50 years old I can honestly say I have never felt better in my life! Thank you Dorothy for all that you do!"*

Lou Anne Monaco
Yoga Teacher, Age 50


*"Dear Dorothy, it was an honor to have you as my Health Coach. Your passion and commitment to your work is inspiring. You immediately pinpointed my frustration, and in a brief period I was able to lose weight in a very natural way. You acted professionally and provided me with clear direction. Also, you have incredible amount of knowledge regarding all aspects of healthy living. I want to let you know that you are very easy to talk to, and that you are a very good listener. You explain things in such a clear manner, and I found your approach to be friendly, compassionate and thoughtful! What I love about you is that you practice what you preach, and your personal story is downright inspiring to me and everyone who knows you. I would recommend you to others who wish to improve their overall health, and I would highly advise them to consider your services."*

Maria Brunetti
Yoga Teacher Age 49


*"At 26 years old, I have been dieting for the past 10 years. I've tried many 'get thin quick' diets and, ultimately, I would fall off the wagon and gained more and more weight. After meeting Dorothy for a consultation, I knew this was something different that I could really benefit from; making a commitment to change my life in just 6 short months. I'm a little over half way through the program and I've already lost over 20 pounds, I'm full of energy, I feel amazing, and the best part is I'm not on a diet. Through Dorothy's guidance, I've gained a new perspective on health and nutrition. This experience has changed my life and I couldn't be more grateful."*

Jolene N. Maggio, MHC-LP

# Acknowledgements

I dedicate this book to my heart's best teachers—my husband Cliff, and my daughters Jessy and Rose.

Thank you Rose Holtermann, you were born on Mother's Day and are a gift that keeps giving. Thank you for the loving bouquet of vegetables you painted for me for the cover.

Thank you Jessy Holtermann you are as beautiful on the inside as on the outside. I am grateful to you and Devin Murphy for producing the video trailer for the book; you both are amazing.

My Mom Marie, thanks for proof reading while bed-bound with your pink cast on your ankle, and putting up with me during this project.

I am so grateful to my sister Patti and my brother Jeff, my big extended family, and my "in laws" (the Holtermann family) with a special loving nod to my mother-in-law, Ethel and my father-in-law, Cliff.

My grandparents, dad, cousins Debra and Carmine, and Jack. I know you are with me all of the time and for all time... but often I just miss you here and now.

I love my teachers. I am grateful for Dr. Cliff Inkles, Dr. Gong, my beloved Jeanette Bronée and Tom Monte. Each of you has created magic and I thank you for holding me and healing me.

I love my community of friends, and I am grateful to Karen Torrone plus the yoga teachers and fellow yogis at 5 Boro. To my courageous Healers' Group brothers and sisters—no words can express my honor to study and grow with each of you.

I love my best friends, Colleen Foley and Ruth Davidson Hahn. Who knew that at 9 years old I would find the perfect friends for all time?

Vito Spatafora, thanks so much for the perfect cover design.

A special word of thanks to Tony Loton, my editor and publishing consultant who went well above the call of duty to push this project over the goal line with great skill and much patience.

# Foreword by Jeanette Bronée

Dorothy came to see me to lose weight, armed with a doctor's note saying that her health was going to cut her life short. She was determined and confused, thinking that she needed to get on a healthy diet, but also convinced that she knew a lot about food and was already doing a good job. Being a foodie, she loved cooking and she grew up in a home of home-cooked food, so in her mind she was all set. As we worked together it became apparent that her food, weight and health issues were far deeper rooted than just bad habits and wrong choices. Realizing that she did not have to be a slave to her medication or a victim of her stress, she stepped away from her existing self-image and took the first steps on her journey of self-discovery with candor and curiosity. This book tells her story.

*** 

Being the courageous and heartful woman that she is, Dorothy set out to learn about herself, her food, and the relationship between the two. Could she learn to love her food and love herself? Her big heart was available to others, but as with many women, she put herself last, and her health was suffering for it. Dorothy's journey to discover her best-thriving and most-nourished self can be regarded as a personal pilgrimage, but one that we all might hope to embark on at some point in our lives. Her story will guide you, inspire you, and give you hope when adversity aims to get the better of you. Dorothy will help you get back up on your feet, and put your next foot forward.

*** 

Join with Dorothy on this journey through the trials and traumas of her life; a story in which she leaves no stone unturned on her road to recovery and self-discovery. She will show you how to move through life with an open and strong heart, with strengthened faith in your body's ability to reverse disease and your own ability to find your way.

\*\*\*

I hope it will inspire you to see how dealing with life's disasters and diseases is more than simply getting through alive, but rather a process of growing into healing that allows us to thrive in spite of it all. Many think of healing as something we do, but Dorothy will show you how it is something that happens when we surrender to ourselves and look inside to find what truly feeds us. Love Food that Loves You Back is a story of falling in love with food, yourself, and others, over and over again, and as you read this book I am sure you will too.

Jeanette Bronée
Founder of Path for Life Self-Nourishment, and author of Eat to Feel Full

# Introduction

Mrs. Esposito lived for 103 years. Yet she lived every year of her life with enviable health and happiness right up until her final days. When she was a mere 86, I asked her what the secret to her robust health was. She told me,

*"Broccoli rabe. I eat broccoli rabe every day; sometimes I eat it two times in one day."*

I asked her why, and she said,

*"Because I love broccoli rabe, and broccoli rabe loves me back."*

The title of this book pays homage to what Mrs. Esposito said.

## Appalling Pandemic

There is an appalling pandemic of diseases spreading around the world and robbing people of their lives—both in terms of quantity (number of years) and quality. These "diet deficiency" diseases include obesity, heart disease, diabetes, arthritis, Alzheimer's, immune disorders and cancer. The sheer number of people directly affected is having an enormous negative impact on nations, their populations, and the resources they rely on. So much "food" is consumed, yet people are starving. And as shocking as the "big picture" may be, we should not forget that every single one of these precious people has a personal tale of tragedy to tell. It is sad that many do not even know it's their food choices making them ill. Some do know, but do not believe that it's *never too late* to do something about it. Some do want to do something about it, but have become trapped on a trail of "one step forward / two steps back" on their journey towards a better body and better health. They blame themselves for their lack of will power—buying into the idea that if they could only fight their cravings, eat less and exercise more, that they would be fit and trim and healthy. They try the plethora of punishing work outs, pills, potions and other supposed panaceas that promise results. Then they get upset when the results don't come; so they give up.

## A Chorus of Disapproval

I wrote this book to contribute my story to a growing chorus of disapproval—about the shocking number of people who are eating themselves into more and more desperate states of disease and despair. You may know one of these people, and you may be one. I was one of them not too long ago.

I invite you to join me in the choir of people singing from the song-sheet of success. People, like me and my family, who have made the Great Escape. Our escape was calamitous and complicated, poignant and perilous, which all went to show that while we can all escape our circumstances... we can't always escape the considerable challenges along the way. But we can face those challenges with faith and fortitude, and recognize them as the disguised gifts they really are; gifts that can propel us to new perspectives on life and love and health. No one would have blamed me for simply giving up and numbing-out with pills and pizza; and for a while... I did. But then I learned (like Mrs. Esposito) to love life by loving the foods that loved me back, and now I'd love to share with you what I learned.

*I was one of the lucky ones. My childhood set the stage for a love of fresh home-cooked whole foods. For decades I loved my food and prepared it with great dedication and devotion for my friends and then young family. I thought that my grandparent-inspired diet was very healthy (if I ignored the fact that all of my grandparents suffered from various diet-based diseases). When healthy food finally healed me, it was tempting to move on with my life and leave the work of spreading the "good news" message to others. But I stumbled upon my life purpose and a calling that could not be ignored; a new vocation to be more vocal and evangelical about health and happiness.*

We cannot stay silent. We cannot be polite. We have huge opposition. The food industry, pharmaceutical industry, the supposed healthcare system, and other "big business" players in Corporate America (and beyond) have left us stuck with systems that do not support our health and happiness. These systems seem too big to battle with, but while money yields power—so does love and compassion. I have learned over and over again that love and compassion can make miracles happen that money just can't buy.

## Sharing My Stories

I love life. I love human beings. I have always been delighted by our love of sharing stories. I especially love food stories, and in particular I adore food stories that expose processed fast food as the villain while hailing healing whole food as the hero. I will be sharing some of my stories in the hope that they may spare you some of some the mistakes I made. Some of the stories will make you laugh, and some may make you cry. I know we all want our lives to be filled with fun stories that have happy endings, not tales of tragedy. The good news, and there's plenty of it, is that mine is a somewhat sad story with a very happy ending.

I have learned that while I could not bypass trauma, I could heal and eventually thrive by adopting life-affirming habits. My favorite foundational life-affirming practice is *learning to love food that loves me back*, and I am a passionate proponent of the idea that *life fully nourished is delicious*. Food profoundly impacts your health, and the food you choose to eat has the most impact on your health—more than anything else you decide to do. I thought I ate a healthy diet. I thought I fed my children healthy food. I thought my parents, and especially my beloved grandparents, ate healthy food. We did get some very important things right about eating, but we also got some very important things very wrong. This became clear to me when my own life fell apart...

## First the Bad News

My life bobbed along the bottom for over a decade as I experienced a seemingly endless litany of tragic life experiences that included dealing with some of my family's debilitating diseases. Then came the devastating disasters of 9/11 and Hurricane Katrina. And finally, the seemingly insurmountable financial fiasco we endured during the recent Great Recession. As my life fell apart, I became hopelessly absorbed with the drama and became completely unaware of my own body and its needs. I ate the wrong food, too much of it, and erratically. I drank too much alcohol. I gained 70lbs. I became dependent on prescription drugs. Internal organs started to fail. My gallbladder was removed. I was stiff and ached and was in constant pain. I became a sad shadow of the young woman I once was. I did not see any way out of this never-ending nightmare.

A visit to my doctor's office sent shockwaves through my system when I was told that I would not live out my lifespan. It proved to be just the jolt I needed to see my life, and open to new possibilities.

## Now the Good News

I made an amazing recovery from over a decade of trauma, and I want to share with you the most important lesson I have learned on the path to recovery: that life fully nourished is delicious.

The crucial first step came when I decided to change and heal my life; when I found that the people who would be pivotal in helping me heal began to appear as if by magic (even if I didn't immediately realize it). I only had to open my eyes and my heart, and my gifted guides would guide me back to health and happiness.

The essence of what I learned is that loving the food I ate – the food that also loved my body – dramatically helped set the stage for healing:

- Eating the food I loved, but which did not love me back, robbed my life of vitality.
- Eating food that loved me, but which I didn't love back, deprived me of the wondrous pleasure and satisfaction and joy of eating—an essential component for a fully nourished, great life.

I wanted the best of both worlds: food that I loved which loved me right back.

I discovered that our planet provides the perfect produce for our perfect health, and what is perfect for our health is also perfect for the health of our planet.. And I'd like to share this good news with the world.

Yes, I have wonderful news. I have important knowledge to share. The great news is that there are a growing number of people lovingly eating themselves into amazing states of health and happiness. They are not *only* preventing disease (and if they only did this then surely it would be enough), they are also healing diseases, recovering from trauma, and fueling wondrous lives of joy and happiness. The food they eat is freeing their bodies from pain and discomfort and is fueling their more fruitful lives. These voices desperately need to get louder.

No one can hate themselves healthy, and the road to wellness is not the path of deprivation and punishment. Eating good food need not be a grim task! You were designed to find great pleasure in good food, and pleasure is actually the surprise secret ingredient of a truly nourishing meal.

## Uniquely You

Although I tell *my* story in this book, it's not all about *me*. It's also about *you*.

You are unique, so the food that loves me might not love you, and vice versa. When you've listened to what I have to say, start listening to your own body, for it will send you the signals to tell you which of the extraordinary assortment of whole foods are best for you.

You are a complex miracle of nature. Each of your trillion cells is a hive of activity, and those cells are in a constant state of organizing and reorganizing with the aim of taking good care of you. We now know that our DNA is not fixed, and its effects can be reformulated by the food we eat and how we live—turning on health-promoting genes and turning off destructive genes. This amazing and powerful news means you have the power to change your destiny in a way not even thought possible just a few short years ago.

It is truly extraordinary that each of us has the power to impact our very being through each and every bite of food we eat. You are what you eat, and you choose the ingredients that make you. Some effects are immediately noticeable, and some are more subtle: your cells are constantly regenerating so that in six years from now you will have a whole new you. You choose the ingredients that will recreate you.

You are wondrous, and I hope my story will help inspire you to lovingly care for yourself so that you can make the most of your miraculous life.

## A Gift from Me to You

As shown on the front cover of this book, I offer you a beautiful symbolic bouquet of vegetables from my heart to yours. If you embrace nature's sacred gift, it will embrace you, and profoundly improve your life and the lives of those you love... forever.

# 1 - You Won't Live Out Your Lifespan

In the fall of 2012 I was badly shaken and forced to face a reality I had long denied.

I was at my doctor's office being analyzed by my "team" of healthcare professionals when it became clear that my weight gain, blood work results, and complaints about various pains were getting progressively worse each visit. They were running out of new prescription drugs to give me, or organs to remove. I was being examined by Keith, my favorite team member, when suddenly he looked me square in the eye and told me bluntly, "Dorothy, you need to do something about your health."

I glanced away, trying to tune him out, ignoring him. I was at the doctor's office, wasn't I? So of course I was taking care of my health! He persisted, and in a more firm tone said, "You need to hear me. You need to listen to me. This is not a joke. This is your life."

I remember looking up, pretending to listen to him, mostly to be polite. I remember thinking—he has nothing to tell me that I do not already know. I was about to make a quip, or find an easy way to bow out of this awkward and highly unusual conversation. However, he did manage to get my attention with his very next sentence. I will never forget hearing these words, and feeling the enveloping fear that they generated in my body.

*"Dorothy, you are not going to live out your lifespan!"*

It was hard to shock me, and I honestly thought I was shockproof, yet...

I thought immediately about my family and what these words would mean to them. I had two beautiful daughters that I loved deeply and who needed me. And I had been married 30 years to my childhood sweetheart and soulmate; the man I treasured and desperately wanted to grow old with. Though not-so-young, I was not-too-old either. Not old enough to hear these words.

My beloved family had been through a lot. It seemed like we had unwittingly managed to purchase front row seats to several of the worst catastrophes of the turn of the 21st century. We were witnesses to the attacks of 9/11 that occurred just blocks from our home, our business, and our daughter's school. A few years later, we fell financial victim to the extraordinarily devastating sequence of multiple hurricanes, including Hurricane Katrina on the Gulf of Mexico which hit our second home and Florida business. In addition, as a family we had suffered from some pretty serious health issues. My husband had been very ill when our children were young, and my oldest daughter had been diagnosed with cystic fibrosis when she turned 10. Each of these things had devastated us. The combination was pitiless yet we continued on, grateful for each other. It was of the utmost importance that we still had one another.

In my heart, I knew, and was ashamed that I had neglected my health. I knew that I was "allowing" my health to be in my blind spot. I had even had a several-year stint smoking cigarettes after having been rather vociferously anti-smoking for decades (especially after my daughter was diagnosed with cystic fibrosis). There was ample evidence that the situation was getting "out of hand" and surely my health was cause for concern, but I was still able to rationalize that – although my health was not great – I hadn't actually gotten quite that bad. I did not believe that I had entered the "die young" department. Dying young at my age meant dying potentially very soon… and I was not ready.

I could not accept Keith's statement as truth. I resisted. I could not fully believe that I was even all that unhealthy. I had thought I was taking pretty good care of myself considering all I had been through. Of course I knew I had to make some improvements to my self-care, but my presumption was that everyone needs to take better care of themselves.

I worked many hours. I knew I worked too many hours. I sat endlessly at the computer, barely moving, sometimes for days on end. I remember feeling almost completely numb. I felt like my head was perched on top of an inanimate pedestal. I made no serious attempt to exercise anymore. Not even stretch. In the past I had at least tried to add in some movement from time to time. I'd join a gym for a few weeks then slowly stop going. I might buy an exercise DVD and give it a go for a few weeks, but nothing really caught on. I had a Raquel Welch exercise tape that was decades old and featured simple 20-minute daily exercises that were easy and fun. I did them occasionally but could not remember the last time I dusted off the tape.

I was always going to get healthy. I hated that I popped pills to feel human enough to function. Once in a while I thought I'd better take better care of myself…soon. Maybe tomorrow…or maybe Monday…or maybe right after the holidays…or when summer was over. The list of future events that would catapult me into the "healthy version" of myself was endless. I thought I knew how to get healthy. Go on an "eat less" diet; join a gym. I was always going to get started. Yet, when the time came, suddenly I was stumped. Why was it always going to be tomorrow? Why did tomorrow never turn into today? I started to think about it. I realized that ignoring my health had been going on for a few decades, and I really did not know how to get "getting healthy" onto the schedule. And year after year, after busy crazy year, there never seemed time for me to do anything any different from what I did the day before. Each day I would work myself into a state of exhaustion or panic. I would do my best to ignore my body completely during the day, and then at some point self-sooth with wine and my perfectly legal prescription medications. I was in a state of trying to survive. But I was not doing a very good job.

Yet, I did not feel that bad. I thought there must be some mistake. Who, me? Unhealthy? No, that is not possible. I was the "know-it-all" woman. I was the wonder woman who cooked with love and passion. I was the woman who ate vegetables. In fact, I had eaten *organic* vegetables for many years! I fed my family well, even when times were hard, which they always seemed to be. We always ate really good fresh food. I had been eating raw milk cheese for a very long time, and buying free range meat for two decades—long before the current popular paleo prescription. .

OK, I knew I had some health issues, but I was convinced that they were due to the traumas. There was nothing I could do about them. I had a few temporary nervous breakdowns, but for darn good reasons, and I always got better. Right? I lived with a lot, and I went through a lot.

I began to reflect. I knew it was not great to need pills and alcohol to "survive", but – considering everything – I was not that bad. I was still cool and intelligent. I knew that at some point I would figure something out. I was troubled. I felt terrible and guilty. I had made some crazy and serious errors of judgment that had compounded our family's problems. But I was back on track and resolving many problems. In the big picture I was just a marvelous, loving, big woman (a little too big at 230lbs for my 5' 1" frame) with a big heart (and, as I recently learned, a big fatty liver).

I continued to think, and I realized it was time for me to recast my story… minus the narrative of endless excuses. Maybe I didn't have all the answers after all. I became present, conscious. I resolved to do more listening and less talking. After all, my physician was a kind and caring person who would not have told me that I was going to "die young" unless he had some solutions.

Although I had long-since lost blind faith in our medical professionals and our "health" care system, and had a preference for alternative "kitchen cabinet" remedies, I did have some residual well-earned respect for the disease detection and management systems of conventional medicine:

*My daughter's diagnosis of cystic fibrosis was detected through a sophisticated DNA test. And her lung therapy vest plus the amazing-though-costly medicines were clearly instrumental in keeping her healthy.*

I had a soft spot for science, and I was certain that your doctor could get you access to that right science if you were persistent… and in my case, admittedly, aggressive and obnoxious. It's the squeaky wheel that gets the grease! Do your own research, and be proactive in helping your physician poke around in their black bags for the right solutions. I believed that if the black bag of tricks didn't already contain the appropriate tool or technique, it soon would do so… thanks to the marvel of modern medicine. I felt confident that all of our maladies – from baldness, to obesity, to cancer, and certainly cystic fibrosis – were on the cusp of being cured with some magic potion, pill, protocol or surgery. Or even better… a natural remedy! I had become accustomed to combatting doctors' slowness and ineptness in sharing the latest and the greatest medical discoveries, but I believed those doctors did offer the best routes to resolution once I had helped steer them in the right direction.

*When my husband got sick, we worked hard and fought hard to get him better. He was a young man and we had just had our second baby. Our oldest daughter was only five. We researched. We battled doctors. At first we used all-natural remedies and healers, but in the end it was conventional medicine (and our insurance, which was a miracle in itself) that rode to the rescue. The surgery was not available in New York, so we flew to San Francisco where a brilliant surgeon had developed the miracle surgery that would heal my husband. It was the cure that we all dream about, and it fit right into my belief system that there was always a "fix." His urinary tract had been damaged in a childhood accident decades earlier. The doctor replaced damaged sections using an amazing internal graft of skin with its own vein that provided the new urinary track with its own blood supply to keep it nice and healthy. The surgery was complicated and daring, but in the end it worked like a charm. My husband used to love to say that the surgery made him "better than new."*

Now it was time for me to work with my doctors and find a cure for myself though I was not sure whether I had faith in my doctor's or myself.

I acted as if I had courage, but the truth is that I felt more than a bit desperate. I felt afraid. It really hit me: my family has been through hell and back. I had not yet "saved us" and I couldn't do so until I saved myself. I had made mistakes that I had to correct. I had made some big nasty soul-crushing decisions. And I had to get into shape and live my life span in order to rebuild our lives and be able to care for others. So it hit me—I had to be healthy for others. Then it hit me again—I also had to be healthy for me. I wanted to be healthy for me. No shame in that.

I realized I did not want to live like this anymore. Who the heck was I? I was a lie. I thought I was taking care of everyone and everything, but it was not true. I cooked. I worked. But in truth I was troubled. Deeply troubled. I failed to see how incompetent I had become—working hard, and achieving less. I took a long hard look at this sad, sick, half dead, mostly lifeless woman who was addicted to prescription drugs and who had become angry with everyone. Everything I did resulted in disaster, but I believed that between disasters I should have figured something out. I was smart, and should have been disaster-proof. Should have seen the solution to every single problem. But I didn't.

Then something happened that changed everything. I felt love for myself. Just a bit, then a bit more, and then a whole lot of love. I thought, "Poor baby, I have to help her!" I began to *rally*. Really. I decided that, HELL, I had no intention of dying young. I would find a fix—not tomorrow, but today. So I said to Keith, my physician's assistant,

*"OK. I am ready. What can we do? I want the newest, latest greatest treatments. I want to get healthy, and I want it NOW! I want to live out my lifespan. I want to be by the side of my beloved husband, beautiful children, and future grandchildren. I*

*am committed, and will do whatever it takes to get my health back on track. Just tell me what to do — today — and I will do it."*

I was waiting for some clear direction, if not exactly a miracle cure.

Keith looked at me, then looked in his desk drawers. I held my breath while he poked around and then pulled something out. He handed me a book. Cool, I thought, a roadmap back to health. But I looked down at it and felt complete despair when I realized the book handed me was a *calorie book*.

I kid you not.

"Are you serious?" I asked.

He was.

I realized he had absolutely no idea as to how to cure me, so I would have to do it myself. I knew it was going to be the project of a lifetime. I was up for a challenge, but where do I begin?

Did I mention that I was morbidly obese, had my gallbladder removed, and my triglycerides were 230? I could not walk up a flight of stairs or walk down the block without the kids having to take turns at "towing" me with their outstretched hands. But since we had previously found a miracle cure for Cliff, and a way to manage Jessy's cystic fibrosis too, then I should be easy enough to fix.

Keith seemed to think that food was the problem, so maybe I could find a food-based solution that would help me reduce my weight and heal my life. But I was still bemused by how a woman with a love of whole foods (passed on from my grandparents), who cooked with a healthy conscience, could end up so sick. I left the doctor's office shaking my head, still uncertain where I had gone wrong.

## 2 – Gorgeous Gardens, Good Food and Gout

I was a lucky child. I was happiest in my grandmothers' kitchens and my grandfathers' gardens. I grew up surrounded by delicious food and lush plants and deep dark dank garden dirt. The kitchens were always brimming with mostly hand-raised and hand-cooked savory food. The aromas are amongst my most vivid and treasured childhood memories.

The simmering rich savory and slightly salty smell of freshly-killed-chicken soup, the smell of fresh pasta drying around the kitchen, and the rich sweet smell of tomato sauce in my Grandmother Rose's kitchen all evoke memories of a safe but adventurous early life, robustly lived. I remember always being surrounded by family during long lingering meals. My grandmother's efforts seemed perfectly "normal" to me, but she worked very hard to put this feast on the table. As soon as one meal was finished, she would say it was "time to start the next meal." This lovingly prepared, slow cooked food was the antithesis of the fast food and TV dinners of the '60s. And I loved it. But it wasn't all roses in Grandma Rose's gourmet garden, as you will read.

## My Grandparents' Garden Gourmet

Moving from Italy to Staten Island, New York in their teens, my grandparents Nick and Rose brought with them a love of food and a joy of gardening and cooking. They worked hard, saved money, and bought a house when my dad, Patsy, and Uncle Benny were young boys. There was a purpose for every patch of their half acre of land, and exploring it was a constant fun adventure. They planted a large garden, raised chickens, and made wine. The wine cellar, dank with a distinct musty smell, was filled with oak barrels and rubber hose for drawing the magical elixir up and out of the barrels and into the carafes for dinner. Long before I learned to like the taste of wine, I loved to linger among the jars of tomatoes, peaches and pears, and my grandfather's specialty – cherry bombs, made from perfectly ripe cherries preserved in brandy – that populated this magical mysterious place.

Grandpa Nick's garden was another magical place, with fairytale twists and turns leading to secret stone tables and built-in benches: perfect places to dine on the garden-grown and apparently ever-lasting (at least until the fall) tomatoes, corn, scallions, peppers, cucumbers, zucchini, pumpkins, chicory, escarole, lettuce, and celery. Small fish ponds were filled with fish… and occasionally my cousin Nicky who seemed to be magnetically attracted to falling in.

The dark damp dirt in Grandpa's garden filled my lungs with earthy aromas plus the not-so-aromatic smell of the pungent cow manure delivered every spring. This was not dead dirt, but was filled with life including earthworms and a multitude of bugs that fascinated me.

My grandfather loved fruit trees and flowers. So did I, particularly the plum, cherry, and my favorite fig trees with their definitive "Italians live here" stamp of authenticity. The garden also featured chestnut, apple, and mulberry trees, and a wonder of a pear tree that grew the three different varieties of pear that Grandpa grafted. The trees created a riotous assortment of colorful flowers in spring, and a cornucopia of fruity natural "sweets" that my grandma would preserve for the cold winter months.

Each year near my birthday in late August, I would get the chance to gorge on the gift of a fresh fig feast when ripe. In the winter those fig trees always looked so comical, covered up in their tar paper winter coat and a "bucket hat".

I was raised a bit wild and free, in complete contrast to today's childhoods that are deprived of unconstrained outdoor adventures in nature. I got into trouble all of the time. I jumped, climbed, and broke off several limbs… fortunately from trees rather than from my own body. I managed to mutilate my grandfather's proudly planted Mimosa that had two large – and very climbable – branches right in front of the house. Crack! That unmistakable crack that sent me running and hiding to escape Grandpa's certain wrath. But wrath turned to relief (for me) when Grandpa Nick dried my tears and whispered,

*"I love my mimosa trees, but I love you so much… so very much more."*

My grandparents made most of their food from scratch: pasta from flour, and sauce from home-grown tomatoes. In the summer, all of the vegetables came from the garden, and freshness was a fanatical pursuit. When the first corn was ready for picking, we would play a game of picking and eating the corn "before it knew it was dead." Grandma shushed us as she prepared the water on the stove; Grandpa shushed us when the water started to boil as we set out to secretly cut the cobs of corn. All so that Grandma could cook the sweet smelling ears just seconds after they were picked. So sweet, yet so crunchy, with each kernel delivering a riot of flavor for us to savor. During our corn crusades, my dad never grew tired of announcing,

*"This corn does not even know it is dead yet!"*

## Foraging for Food

My dad and his family were wild food foragers. We ate wild dandelions (which we called "circoria") with great fervor in spring. I remember the shocked expression on my girlfriend Ruth's face when she walked into a frenzied feast in my Mom's kitchen one spring day and exclaimed, "You guys eat *grass. GROSS!*" As a young dancer (later a founding member of the Mark Morris Dance Company), Ruth was perpetually hungry and her curiosity was peaked. So of course she had to try some, even though my constantly comedic father tried to playfully dissuade her by pretending to sneeze into the rapidly disappearing bowl of greens. Undeterred, she dug her fingers in to try one. "WOW!" she exclaimed, "these *weeds* are so delicious. I want more!"

*Though we knew we felt great after eating them, and we madly enjoyed them, we did not know or even think that these "weeds" might also be packed with healthy micronutrients, vitamins and minerals.*

One day, my then-boyfriend Cliff and I we were driving by Richmondtown when I barely spotted my grandmother Rose and her sister Edith bending over in the grass on the roadside, sporting kerchiefs to cover their heads and most of their faces. I shouted out, and they held their heads down, trying not to acknowledge me before waving me on. This strange behavior can be explained with a little history:

*My now-husband Cliff's German family had a large bakery originally built in old Richmondtown. It was so beloved that he was deemed quite the "catch", and my family thought I was marrying into Staten Island royalty.*

With this in mind, my aunt's strange behavior seemed not so strange when she later explained to me,

*"Dorothy when we wear kerchiefs in our hair like that, we do not want to be recognized. We are embarrassed."*

Well, they may have been embarrassed, but my soon-to-be foodie husband and I thought that it was awesome for them to be foraging for wild food.

Many years later, I was walking with my dad in my lovely second home town on the Gulf of Mexico in Seaside, Florida. An older gentleman with plaid shorts suddenly presented me with a challenge as we walked past the Italian inspired garden of the town's founding couple, Robert and Daryl Davis. In his Brooklyn Italian accent, the old man said, "Hey, goylie, I will give ya a million bucks if ya can tell me what these are!" Without missing a beat I told him, "Oh them. They're cicoria". "You gotta be kiddin me!" he said, "I wouldda given ya a million bucks jus ta know they w' dandelions. Now I owe ya 2 million bucks cus ya knew they were cicoria." We did not stop to chat with him, and enjoyed leaving him scratching his head at the thought that in the middle of the *panhandle* of Florida a young woman had known and said the Italian name for dandelions—complete with a New York accent!

\*\*\*

## Recipe for Dandelion Salad

Here is my recipe for dandelion (cicoria or in an Italian NY accent "chigoidia") salad (serves 2):

- 4 cups of dandelions (best wild in spring when small and tender or chopped if larger).
- 2 cloves of garlic.
- 3 tablespoons of extra virgin olive oil.
- 1 tablespoon of red wine vinegar.
- Sea salt.

Crush the garlic and let rest in olive oil and vinegar on the bottom of your salad bowl while you clean and prepare the greens and then mix salad.

*(For crazy fun I recently added some chopped fresh figs, which combined two of my favorite foods in the world and made an interesting contrast of bitter and sweet)*

\*\*\*

In the fall, my dad and my brother Jeff would feed our family's passion for wild mushrooms by foraging the then-vast tracks of natural land on Staten Island as early as 4am on dark damp rainy mornings. The "hen of the wood" mushrooms – which we called "mamma la fungie," but which most people now call "maitake" as a nod to the Japanese who cultivate them – could be as large as a small child. My nephew Michael, who continues the tradition to this day, recently foraged one the size of our outdoor table-for-six. These delicious magical mushrooms are also magically healthy, with new studies showing that they can reduce blood sugar and provide anti-cancer immune support. No wonder the

Japanese call them the dancing mushrooms (because people dance when they find them). Now that I know the Japanese tradition, I also dance.

***

## Recipe for Wild Mushroom Sauté

Here is my recipe for wild mushroom sauté (which can be adapted for just about any vegetable):

- 2 cups of mushrooms (maitake, shitake, oyster. Even simple white buttons will do you some good but disappoint your taste buds.)
- 2 cloves of garlic, crushed and chopped.
- Hot red pepper flakes.
- 3 tablespoons of extra virgin olive oil (unfiltered and organic if available).
- Sea salt.

Towel clean your mushrooms unless they are wild (and you have picked them with someone who knows what they are doing!). Then seriously clean by soaking and rinsing in water several times to make certain you will not be ingesting some extra squiggly protein; and towel dry.

Heat heavy pan (I use cast iron) on high for a few minutes. Lower heat to medium and add garlic, red hot crushed pepper to taste, and – in a minute more – the mushrooms.

Push the mushrooms around in the pan with a wooden spoon. Mushrooms will give up a bit of moisture, but try to get the mushrooms to brown just a bit.

Add sea salt to taste.

Eat. And dance again.

***

## Dad, the Deer Hunter

My dad was a man's man. Sandlot football hero, fisherman, baseball player, and the affable and always fun owner / bartender of the Oak Villa restaurant.

For decades he was the head hunter at the hunting club house we call called "The Ponderosa." And with his 8pt dear head hung above the dining table which he said would only be displaced when someone else caught a deer with a bigger rack. When the fall came he would hold a free venison feast at our restaurant featuring the meat he killed. In the spring he would host a free fish feast with the fish he caught. No one knew that he did not actually eat the fresh-killed meat or fish, but he did not waste it either.

Dad owned a three-wheeled Daihatsu from Japan, which my grandpa Carmine had used when buying fish in the Fulton fish market in Manhattan. My dad liked to make me laugh by occasionally driving it up on the sidewalk with me on board. He liked to beep and say hello to imaginary people. He was generous to a fault—always wanting to pick up restaurant tabs for everyone. Everyone loved Patsy (that's my dad) but my mom and we kids worshipped him.

At 4'6" it was Grandma Rose – rather than  Grandpa Nick, or her sons, my dad or Uncle Benny – who was the unlikely real killer in the family. She killed chickens and rabbits for meat, and she killed possums for raiding her vegetable garden. Grandma's last "chicken kill" became family lore:

*My dad and brother Jeff found a half-dead scrawny chicken on a construction job site, and brought it home to my now-infirm grandma as a joke. That night Jeff dreamt a dream that featured muffled clucking and screeching, and woke up to the distinct smell of chicken soup… it wasn't a dream. Chicken soup was on Grandma's menu that morning.*

My sister Patti and I lived down the block from Grandma. One morning, Patti woke up to find a huge possum at the foot of our basement steps. She was home alone with her three children and called our "family possum expert" to find out what to do. Grandma told her not to worry, and that she would arrange to have the possum captured. I was upstairs and could see my 82-year-old grandma casually walking down the street dragging a big baseball bat behind her. How curious, I thought, having no idea about my sister's dilemma. Suddenly I hear the BAM-BAM-BAM accompanied by the sound of Patti and her kids all screaming and crying. Grandma had her hand on her heart, and was breathing heavily, but the possum was as dead as dead can be. I was furious,

*"Are you guys all crazy? You know that the score came too close for comfort: Humans—1, Possums—1?"*

The final kill story was dubbed the "thwarted kill", and it happened in our Pocono Mountain home. Grandma and I were on the deck overlooking our property filled with beautiful white birch trees. Suddenly a large and loud flock of wild turkeys decided to pay us a visit, delighting me and all of my children. Wild turkeys were always my favorite and I found their gaggling so joyfully comical. Grandma was tugging on my shirt and asked me to bend down so she could whisper into my ear "Go open the garage door, but very quietly." It seemed an odd request, so I asked her why. Then I saw the killer glint in her eyes. We were all seeing and delighting in the festive live turkey parade… but Grandma was seeing roasts, drumsticks and a great opportunity for some free meat. I yelled at her, "No, Grandma, NO!"

## My More Modern Maternal Grandparents, and Mom

My maternal grandparents were more "modern," but every bit as fun and seemingly exotic. My grandfather, Carmine, was a longshoreman with a taste for international fruit and delicacies including "Chinese apples" (which are pomegranates to you and me). These were eaten with ceremony, and with my namesake Grandma Dorothy's entire living room covered with newspaper to keep it pristine. In addition to the persimmons, kiwis, and different colored bananas, Grandpa also brought home all kinds of foreign spices which were perfect for show-and-tell in school. My German grandma was taught to cook by her Italian mother-in-law, but complemented the Italian cuisine with her "cute little" meat roasts. Whatever my Grandmother Dorothy made was utterly and absolutely delicious. She made the best French fries from freshly cut potatoes fried in fine olive oil. My grandmother would accommodate my grandfather's curiosity for trying new delicacies even though they made her squeamish. When my grandfather brought home frog legs; Grandma would cook them. When he brought home wild duck or goose; Grandma would cook them. Then Grandma Dorothy would immediately discard the cooking pan, right out the window into the alley way.

I absolutely believed that my grandparents' own-grown home-cooked food *did us good* as well as *tasted good*, and it took decades for me to question this. Clearly *some of the food we loved, loved us back*, yet something was wrong. Some of the food was making us sick, as you will soon see.

My own mother cooked in the more modern sixties style, with meat and potatoes and more of a focus on fast food. Not as bad as many of my friends who were consuming canned cuisine and "TV dinners" that lacked even the single vegetable component – usually corn or peas, but always salad – that complemented Mom's freshly made food. We ate lots of red meat, and enjoyed lots of bread, often dunked in the juices from our blood-red steaks. We loved potatoes, freshly mashed, and not the freeze-dried food prepared by some of my friends parents.

The main difference between my parents' and grandparents' eating habits was the fanfare that accompanied my grandparents' faire. While both of my grandfathers loved their vegetables, we relegated vegetables to the status of a "side dish" with meat, fish or pasta as the centerpiece of every meal. In Italian, vegetables are called "I contorni" and are meant to *round out or contour a meal.*

Since my mom worked, she did use some canned food and Campbell's soups for convenience. And she switched from fresh butter to modern margarine to help improve my dad's heart health… without realizing that this industry-introduced panacea would turn out to be more deadly than the food it was replacing. We ate hot dogs. We gorged on grilled meats. We loved meat. And bread. And pasta.

My Mom was proud that she did not buy much "junk" food, but she had no fear of chemical ingredients and easily succumbed to any fad that she believed would be healthier for her husband and kids. Like so many other housewives, she declared war on fat by buying "fat free" foods without realizing that the real enemy might be the sugar that was used in increasing amounts to fill the hole left by the flavorsome fat. Like the artificial flavors that she also ignored, sugar made food taste good. And if it tasted good, it was probably doing us good, or so she thought.

Compared with our other staple foods – potato chips and my mom's favorite Cheez-Its – I actually thought that my grandparent's food was better tasting, more interesting, and more fun to eat. And I was lucky to eat regularly at both grandparents' households, often once or twice a week. However, I thought my mom cooked better than my friends' mothers did, and I thought I was very lucky to eat her food. We ate out at real restaurants—fresh seafood, and surf 'n' turf. We avoided McDonald's for reasons of good taste rather than good health, so we went to Bacci's (a wonderful little restaurant) for our very big burgers. And French fries formed from fresh potatoes. And massive chocolate milkshakes.

Since my parents and grandparents Carmine and Dorothy had owned and operated a restaurant together, much of my childhood was focused on food. I worked in the restaurant between the ages of 9 and 17, and my last position there was as Assistant Chef. I did do a day as Head Chef on a single Sunday before the restaurant was sold, and my dad teased me that it was my cooking which made him have to sell. Our food was good, but not as good as the Italian food that we enjoyed at home and which (ironically) would not have been appreciated by the restaurant visitors of the 1960s.

## Family Health Matters

My grandparents had been poor as children, and they could each remember when there was not enough food to eat. They were delighted that their new country had plenty of everything, and they enjoyed it without restraint. They ate too much. To be hungry was an emergency. As a kid, if you told my Grandmother Rose you were hungry, it could be 2 o'clock in the morning and the kitchen would fly open for some pastina and butter... or anything else you might want her to cook. She was proud of her 24/7 open kitchen.

On Sunday there was course after course until the men (especially) of the family fell to the floor, or onto the sofa, with their top pant buttons undone in order to breathe better. The couch looked like a crime scene, and it was scary. My siblings and cousins and I were lucky enough to escape into the woods with Grandma, on our nature hikes outside her garden. We hunted painted turtles, and counted the squares on their backs to determine their ages. We picked wild flowers for our mothers, Marie and Lydia. Grandma handed out generous hunks of Hershey milk chocolate for us to gobble down. She loved us, and we loved her back.

Much of what Grandma did was focused on food. If you opened your mouth in her garden, it just might get filled with a meatball. If you were thin like my poor cousin Debbie, Grandma would be on a mission to plump you up. Come to think of it, thin or fat, we were all very lovingly *force fed*. Food would be thrown into us rather than being thrown out with the garbage, even though the garbage might have been the better option. My poor easy-going and eager-to-please sister Patti became overweight and began a lifelong obesity battle.

I noticed my grandparents lived with a lot of discomfort, but I comforted myself with the knowledge that "it was normal," or with the fact that my Grandpa Nick – to my young eyes, at least – was an old man when he died of cancer at the not-so-ripe old age of only 63. We always blamed the Park's Department where he worked and where he could have been exposed to chemicals while on duty, but there were plenty of signs that his diet was the real problem. He had always been overweight. He suffered horrifically and frequently from gout, and I remember his poor big toe looking like it was one of his cherry bombs: big and bright red. His diet did not seem deficient in fruit and vegetables, but these were overly complemented with pasta and bread and chocolate and brandy and beer and wine.

Grandma Rose was also overweight, with 130lbs of weight supported by her tiny 4'6" frame. She suffered from arthritis from her early fifties, and got so desperate for pain relief that she submitted herself to experimental gold injections which seemed to help her arthritis but probably damaged her heart. She developed heart disease, had several life-limiting heart attacks, and finally died of a stroke at age 84.

Grandma Dorothy died more recently of Alzheimer's disease, although in truth she died to us a decade earlier when she was robbed of her joyful personality and then any knowledge of any of us. She had been overweight as long as I can remember and had suffered terribly from arthritis—barely being able to walk in her late fifties when she and grandpa accompanied my husband (poor man) and me to Europe on our honeymoon. She got colon cancer at sixty, but was philosophical about the fact that it was all part of life for people to suffer increasing illness from their 50s and 60s onwards. What she didn't realize is that it didn't have to be this way, and that her diet was a major contributor to these conditions. She ate Uneeda biscuits and butter every day for breakfast, and even fed the same to her beloved poodle, Charlie.

*"You feed your dog biscuits and coffee, Grandma?"* I asked.

*"But Charlie loves his breakfast"* she said somewhat defensively.

No wonder Charlie got obese, had arthritis, and was *nervous*.

Although she ate some vegetables and loved to prepare greens for my grandfather, Grandma Dorothy also loved pasta and a generous amount of meat. She liked pastry and cheeses, and she could eat three hotdogs in a single sitting. All washed down with dry red wine and Scotch whisky. She suffered at night, and called her bed her torture chamber. But to me she was a food goddess. When she went into the hospital for knee replacements and my grandfather was forced to eat my food – reluctantly – he astonished me by saying "It almost takes like Grandma made it. You cook the most like Grandma." I felt like I had won the Academy Award of cooking, because, like I said, I regarded Grandma as a gastronomic goddess and Grandpa was the pickiest eater I knew.

Grandpa Carmine was thin. He lost most of his stomach in his forties from an ulcer operation. He liked his vodka and tonic… a little too much. He also liked seafood, vegetables and fruit. He did headstands and was playful and fun. He enjoyed inventing imaginary people with fantastic names to torment my cousins as children. He was very active and enjoyed gardening, especially when he retired and created a mini farm in Florida. Although unhealthy as a young man, he remained fairly healthy into his seventies. Having been a smoker from his early days, he ended his days – suddenly, from lung cancer – while on dialysis for failing kidneys.

## Moving Beyond Blind Belief

I admired my grandparents and am so grateful for the love of home cooked meals and fresh local whole food that they taught me to prepare, appreciate and enjoy. They raised chickens, and they highly valued fresh-killed meat and fresh eggs. We ate venison from the hunters as often as possible. So far so good, but we also ate conventionally raised red meat and pork, and enjoyed our cured prosciutto, pepperoni and other dried sausages.

We also enjoyed seafood. Grandpa Carmine went to the Fulton fish market to buy fish for the restaurant, and brought us home some wonderful fresh fish that we all enjoyed. We ate wild caught seafood, especially when my dad met his friend Mimi to pull fresh crabs straight from the sea on the New Jersey shoreline at the end of summer each year. Despite working fulltime jobs (even my grandmothers), my grandparents always managed to grow and prepare amazing slow-cooked food. They inspired me to do the same: cook up whole food with fanfare while holding down a job. In short, I thought that my grandparents' diets were great examples of how to eat and feed your family.

We ate one or two servings each of fruit and vegetables every day—far more than our friends who didn't enjoy the luxury of fresh food rather than canned or frozen. We may not have fully realized that "fresh is best" from a health perspective, but out taste buds told us that wild foraged food was tastier than the pale pink tomatoes shipped in from afar. The food that we loved, loved us back. Grandma Rose never had to persuade us to gobble up our greens, and she was far more likely to scold us to finish our "cha chi"—Grandma Rose's childish Italian slang for meat. That proved to be a serious problem.

While we were pretty judgmental about the "crappy" food other people in our community ate, we never considered the potential correlation between my grandparents' diets and their diseases. We never would have dreamed that our food would be deemed unhealthy just a few decades later, or that my grandparents' food rather than theirs ages caused their painful and debilitating diseases. To be fair, alcohol was singled out as a potential demon drink, but the enjoyment always seemed to outweigh the potential health risks.

I now know that the bread and pasta, and other white flour products that our family consumed in abundance, were quickly converted to sugar once consumed. But were worse than sugar itself due to the higher glycemic index (the sugar impact). We ate cake, cookies, and milk chocolate, and we put anisette in our black "demitasse" coffee. The worst culprit was Grandma Rose's fresh fried dough, covered in sugar, which was my favorite desert. Grandma Rose was never diagnosed with diabetes, luckily, unlike her mother and sister who both suffered from the disease. On the savory side, her "suicide sauce" (my dad's words, due to his inevitable incidental indigestion) was filled with meat. Pigs' feet, sausage, meatballs, pork ribs and beef ribs all went into Grandma Rose's Sunday sauce, and we knew that the sauce was ready when there was an inch of fat floating on top of the slow cooked tomatoes (loaded with healthy lycopene, but a nightshade vegetable that can aggravate arthritis).

I continued with the same beliefs, without much contemplation, until my own family started to become ill. Even as "fast food" became all the rage, we remained committed to our traditional diet, without realizing how far it had veered from the authentic Italian diet. When my Grandmother Rose took my cousin Diane and me to Italy in our teens, we discovered just how Americanized out Italian cuisine had become... with more meat and much bigger portions. *We loved our food*, but it *did not love us back.*

## 3 – Happy Days, Happy Meals and Hereditary Health

While I was away at college, I began to realize how my notion of myself was so intimately connected with my notion of food. This chapter is all about my "Happy Days" cooking at college, the "Happy Meals" that should have been called SAD (as in the Standard American Diet), and the "Heredity Health" issues that I assumed I had inherited from my grandparents. Plus as few more assorted stories along the way.

## College Chef

I was only 17 when I went away to college at Stony Brook University. It made me both homesick (missing my family) and food-sick (because I could not consume the food they served in the college cafeteria). My homesickness was addressed by my lovely Aunt Catherine who had each of her five children mail me weekly letters and cards to comfort me. My food-sickness was combatted by me learning to greatly expand my cooking skills out of sheer necessity. As a freshman, I was mandated to be on the food plan. I could not believe that people could eat such poorly prepared food, I thought it was tragic, and I remember calling my mother:

*"Mommy, there is no food here! It is not real food. I cannot eat it!"*

I constantly asked my classmates how they could bear to eat such terrible food. People thought I was funny, but I was *oh-so serious*.

After a few weeks of eating in the cafeteria, it dawned on me that I could bypass the requirement of eating in the cafeteria by buying as much raw cafeteria food as I could and bringing it back to my dorm room to cook it myself. I convinced my roommates to do the same. We would supplement the cafeteria food (mostly meat) with fresh vegetables from the supermarket. On Fridays the cafeteria served steak, and – to the consternation of the kitchen staff – we would order the steak *raw* (not merely *rare*) to cook back at base camp. Our dorm rooms did not have kitchens, so we made our own kitchen from brought-in refrigerators, hot plates and large toaster ovens. My "suite" mates brought in all kinds of pots and pans that had formed the flotsam and jetsam of their parents' kitchens—dull knives and mismatched everything. Cooking in a "kitchen" equipped with such a limited array of appliances presented a number of cooking challenges, but I eagerly accepted the challenges and I actually thought of my patched-together kitchen as having a certain charm. I set out to develop more modern versions of my grandparents' recipes, and I even bought New York Times food critic Craig Claiborne's International Cookbook in an attempt to broaden my culinary horizons.

We created our own meal plan, and I was soon cooking up a storm every night for ten students—my new, big family. I cooked every night, it seemed using every single pot and pan, and thankfully I never had to do the dishes in the tiny bathroom sinks. Although I must say so myself, my food was delicious and I became very popular and a bit of a food prima donna. One night when I was making ravioli, my roommate came back from the supermarket with canned Chef Boyardee ravioli rather than the ingredients I had put on the shopping list for my fresh tomato sauce and frozen freshly-made raviolis. She thought she was doing me a favor, buying the already prepared version that she had been eating at home. I threw such a fit that she felt forced to drive forty minutes back to the store to get the ingredients I told her that I absolutely needed.

I was proud of myself. I thought there was no one at Stony Brook who ate as deliciously and healthily as the kids I cooked for every night. They bragged to their mothers about me, and people would come in to see if it the rumors were true. We had a waiting list for other students who wanted to join my meal plan.

## Health Food or Horse Feed?

I cared about health, and took many trips to the Port Jefferson health store where I loved the classes but not the food. I thought the health food tasted heavy and dull, and I did not like the smells that could not compare with the smells coming from my dorm room… let alone from my grandmothers' kitchens. It might have loved my body, but I had no love for the health food of the 1970s. The vegetables were limp, and the grains tasted like cardboard. I remember saying that the food should be served in a bucket to horses.

My roommates were willing diners in my experimental kitchen. When not relying on my cookbook, I'd call up Grandma Dorothy to ask:

*"Grandma, how did you make pulpo?" (octopus)*

*"Grandma, how did you get your turkey stuffing to stay so firm?"*

Now the bad news. I entered college weighing 115lbs and exited weighing 135. A little chubby… but very popular, happy, and (I believed) still quite healthy.

## Raising Children

When I started to cook for my husband and children, I knew a lot about food. I thought I knew *everything* about food, and loved to lecture people quite convinced that I was an expert. I took great delight in the delusion of being one of the healthiest and best home cooks in the world. I was a food snob, a preacher, and a pain in the ass who turned my nose up at anything processed.

I had upgraded many ingredients from my college days to increase the nutrition in the food.

My family's health issues provided me with the passion to feed them the healthiest food I could find, using increased information from the books and magazines I believed in—to feed us *food that loved us back.*

I remember looking at the boxes of garbage on the supermarket shelves with despair; aisle after aisle of prepared foods that needed no refrigeration. Boxes and bags of lifeless fake ingredients and "designed' food; designed to trick our senses into thinking we were eating real food. But deep down, some of us knew that this culinary crap was slowly sickening us and our children. Surely this couldn't last long, and people would "wake up" to the fact that this food was unhealthy and did not even taste good. But I too *occasionally* made the mistake that my grandparents made: if food *tasted good*, I ate it.

Most times, I never bought boxed food before fully analyzing the ingredients list, which led to the following conversation with my young daughter Jessy:

*"Why are you reading those boxes, Mommy?"*

*"Mommy is trying to find food that doesn't have artificial colors and flavors."*

*"What are artificial colors and flavors, Mommy?"*

*"Not real food."*

*"You mean like rocks? Oh Mommy, everyone knows you only put real food in your mouth."*

That's my girl! She will stop the madness, and the next generation won't put up with the poison in our foods. I'll raise her to relish real food, like my grandparents did with me.

That conversation with my toddler happened over *20 years ago*, and not that much has changed since then. The food industry tricks may have changed – such as replacing "unhealthy" fat in food with equally unhealthy sugar and salt – but we're still being fooled about food. If the fat won't kill you anymore (but don't count on it) the sugar and salt surely will.

## Food Tricks and Toddlers

Big business is in the business of increasing profits rather than improving our health: billions of dollars being invested in advertising or wasted on pointless *product development*; government subsidies spent on tricking you into eating fake food. But no one is actually *forcing* you into the fake food fantasy, so where's the harm in this merely passive poisoning?

In fact, the food factories are busy developing evermore innovative food products to help us overcome the clinical conditions we previously never knew we had: such as creating processed food with the gluten taken out. So now we can buy fake factory food that is actually healthy. Or is it?

*The experiment to create human food in a factory rather than on the farm has failed, and it's time to stop paying money to poison our populous and instead use all government subsidies to support farmers growing organic food (medicine). Then our food might love us back.*

I first became aware that the food raised and grown in America was not the best it could be while on vacation in Europe.

When Jessy was a baby, we took my 11-year old nephew Christopher to Holland with us on vacation. Christopher was a picky eater and on the airplane he carefully counted the food he would eat. "I eat eight things: chicken, potatoes, broccoli, macaroni, corn, spinach, bread, and carrots. And that is it." Each night we would order him the simplest chicken dish on the menu. He would swoon, he would swear "THIS is the BEST meal I ever ate." Night after night after night the same accolade after his meal. We finally started to taste what we presumed was a pretty bland meal only to discover that he was quite right. His simple roasted chicken was absolutely amazing. This made me question why the meat in America tasted so insipid in comparison. I discovered to my surprise and sadness that our meat was being raised in appalling conditions and it was filled with antibiotics. Europe remained traditional in raising meat, and for health reasons banned the import of USA produced meat. That shocking revelation made me decide to do my best to avoid eating or feeding my family American conventionally raised meat.

After returning from Europe, I looked to buy healthier, free-range meats. This became easier when we moved to Manhattan. My favorite story about Rose (my youngest daughter) is the one in which we were shopping in Balducci's, a gourmet food store that sold venison and wild game.

*"What would you like for dinner, honey? Ostrich, venison, or buffalo?"*

While sitting in her stroller sucking her thumb (which she claimed tasted of broccoli-probably to insure that she could indulge her habit), she said,

*"I want buffalo mommy, it's my favorite."*

A woman waiting at the counter looked around aghast,

*"Seriously. I mean, seriously. Are we being filmed? Is this a joke? Or does your child really eat buffalo?"*

I also really understood that the children had to eat vegetables daily, so I developed many great strategies to help them wittingly or unwittingly chomp them down. Rose had asked Cliff, my husband, if she could become a vegetarian. But when not sucking on her broccoli-flavored thumb, we noticed that she ate ninety percent of her calories in pasta, butter and cheese… with only an occasional raw carrot, or her vegetable-obsession-of-the-month, or (most interesting of all) jicama!, Cliff told Rose,

*"No, you cannot be a vegetarian until you eat VEGETABLES! You cannot be a vegetarian if just want to be a noodle head."*

The realization that she ate so few vegetables inspired me to double my efforts. One of my best and most fun strategies for tricking my children into eating more vegetables was the "goodies salad" strategy that worked like a charm every time. Every night I would prepare the salad with chopped-up add-ins like olives, carrots, jicama, avocado, peppers and celery. The greens were the salad, and all the other things were the "goodies" which I hid under the lettuce leaves. I would tell the girls that they could only have a few of these goodies before Daddy came home, and of course I found that they would all be gone before Dad came through the door.

\*\*\*

## Recipe for Goodies Salad

Here is the recipe for my goodies salad (with my secret ingredient—tamari):

The idea is to add lots of color and lots of flavor to make these veggie offerings very appealing. Experiment, have fun, and have the kids pick out 'goodies" when shopping. Be confident and *tricky,* and *insist* that they must share... because these are *goodies!* Some good choices of goodies include...

- Olives of any kind or color, but black seem to be the most popular with kids.
- Cucumbers; try to get the thin skinned.
- Red or yellow peppers.
- Carrots raw or lightly steamed (if you see any red carrots, grab them, because they are filled with even more antioxidants and are yummy).
- Artichoke hearts or bottoms (even lowly canned, frozen or jarred are filled with nutrition and fiber).
- Cruciferous broccoli or cauliflower, lightly steamed. Both are nutritional powerhouses, and cauliflower is one exception to the "no white food" rule.
- Steamed string beans.
- Chunks of raw cabbage (red is best).
- Radishes—daikon and jicama Rose's oddball favorite (another exception to the no white food rule)

- Avocado (very popular in my house too-and crazy good for everyone)

Cover with greens. Not too many dark greens for kids, but mix up like a spring salad.

Dressing—I like a 3-part extra virgin olive oil / 1-part balsamic dressing, crushed garlic and my magical and not-so-Italian ingredient: the amazing and lovely tamari Japanese sauce, similar to soy but with a more complex flavor. I buy the wheat-free low sodium version and use in salad to replace sea salt.

Experiment! My kids liked their salad without dressing when they were young, and might instead dunk it in their glass of water.

*** 

While I wasn't exactly proud of my subterfuge, I figured that all was fair in love (for food) and war. And my children did eat a massive amount of vegetables this way. They ate seaweed under the guise of "Mermaid salad", safe in the knowledge that it would help them sing like Ariel, their favorite Disney character.

## My Children Charm Me with Chocolate

My clever children also learned a few food tricks of their own. One Saturday afternoon after their weekly acting lesson in SoHo, I took my daughters Jessy and Rose with my niece Marie food shopping in Gourmet Garage. I was chatting away with them in the store without realizing that no one was answering me. Calm at first, I panicked when I realized they were not anywhere in the store any more. I ran out of the store, leaving my shopping cart behind, and found them all sitting nicely together on a bench on the sidewalk in front of the store. But I was furious.

*"You KNOW you are not to leave the store without me. Are you all CRAZY? Hmmm…hmmmmm oh… well at least you're all OK. Please don't do it again, my sweethearts."*

A man on the next bench began to laugh.

*"You don't even know what just happened. Your daughter changed you with a chocolate."*

Rose had climbed on the bench, quickly unwrapped a Ghirardelli chocolate, and had slipped it into my screaming mouth. And I stopped screaming—my fiery temper instantly extinguished.

This is an amazing example of the power of food. It demonstrates how easy it can be to turn to food to improve mood, and why we need self-compassion to shift our choices and change our habits.

## Healthy and Happy, not SAD

Jessy's health was amazing considering she had cystic fibrosis. She never missed school, and even more extraordinary, she never went to the hospital. But my younger daughter Rose's health was nothing short of miraculous. Rose was never ill for more than an hour or two, and never took antibiotics… ever. No earaches, no sore throats, and – unlike her friends – no ever-present pink bottle of amoxicillin in the refrigerator throughout the winter. She never had a "sick" visit to the doctor. It took over an hour for the nurse to find Rose's health records when she needed them for High School. The nurse said she had never seen such a thin record. She even wondered if Rose had a different doctor somewhere.

*I took massive pride in the fact that we only served healthy food at home, and my children were all models of great health because of it.*

We realized how far we had veered from the "Standard American Diet" (which was "SAD" by name and "SAD" by nature) when we were visited by our friends Chris and Jeff from Alabama. They came into our home tired from their long trip.

*"Do you have a Coke?"*

*"I'm sorry, we do not drink soda."*

So I offered them flavored water instead.

"Do you have coffee?"

*"No, we have no coffee, but I can offer you dandelion tea."*

They accepted it reluctantly.

*"Could we have some milk and sugar?"*

*"Well, I can offer you soy milk and organic honey."*

You get the idea. And so did they, when they finally exploded with,

*"Where the heck are we?! Is this still America?!"*

What can be more modern-American than the McDonald's golden arches? One day we were driving in our tan Mitsubishi Galant from Manhattan to Sugar Hill, New Hampshire to visit with our best friends Colleen and Jack. It was a long drive and I had no time to pack much food before we set out, so we were going to stop midway to eat a meal. We were all pretty hungry, and the kids were whining when we started to look for a place to eat. Our daughter Rose lit up with a glimmer of hope when she saw those famous golden arches.

*"Please, oh please Daddy. Can we? Can we eat there just this once?"*

Cliff calmly countered that we would go into a town to find a restaurant.

Rose got mad, got furious, and continued complaining,

*"Why can't we eat at McDonald's? Everyone eats at McDonald's! Seriously Daddy, it's like we are not even Americans!"*

Cliff just simply said,

*"Sorry Rose. . We are Americans and we are proud to be Americans who eat real food."*

Yes, we resisted fast food as much as we could, and did a good job of it. I believe this was also a primary reason why our kids' health was so good.

The only time I remember taking my older daughter Jessy to McDonald's was when she was invited to a birthday party at around age 4. She was elated. She could barely wait. The golden arches beckoned her, and she could not believe her good fortune—that her friend was having a birthday party there AND her mom and dad were letting her go to it! She had heard the amazing rumors that this restaurant gave you a toy with every meal, which seemed too good to be true.

*"Wow, Mommy, I cannot wait to go, you get real toys with your meal!"*

The truth was that the children got *real toys* but *not real food*. She ordered a "Happy Meal" with a hamburger, and delighted me when she was not happy. She took the gray listless burger from the bun and asked me what it was.

*"It is meat, honey."*

She held it between her fingers, looking at it intently, and kind of wiggled it. Then she smelled it.

*"It doesn't look like meat, Mommy. It doesn't smell like meat, Mommy. No Mommy… really, what is it?"*

I looked at it.

*"Honestly, Jess, I just do not know."*

## Meeting My Husband's Demands

Husbands can be very demanding of their wives. Some husbands demand sex every evening, and some demand beer. My husband, too, was very demanding... but in a very different way. He demanded vegetables, and was effectively a veggieholic! Sometimes he drove me crazy with how many vegetables he wanted to eat each evening. He would balk at broccoli when presented as a single spear, and would scream...

*"This is not a serving of vegetables, this is garnish! I want my OWN head of broccoli! A whole head to myself!"*

I would joke,

*"Some woman marry alcoholics or gamblers, and apparently I married a veggieholic. I guess that's not so bad."*

I would chop-chop-chop. He would chomp-chomp-chomp. He stayed trim. He got healthier and healthier after years of illness. But where he led, I did not follow, and sadly it showed.

## Wining, Dining, with the World on the Doorstep

I read about food all of the time, and I was pleased beyond words when my grandparents' Mediterranean diet was lauded for being so healthy despite the plethora of pasta and bread (and admittedly healthy vegetables and olive oil). I felt vindicated that I had never fallen for the alternative "fat free" processed products mantra.

I did know our diets were not perfect. We ate a lot of "healthy" cookies and cakes, and drank a little (arguably a lot) too much wine. My husband and I, not the children, you understand. And we enjoyed our Armagnac, just to be civilized. Not perfect, I know, but still much better than how most people ate.

We didn't just drink our wine; as true "foodies" we studied it and made notes in our wine journals. My brother and his friends would entertain themselves by reading out tasting notes when they were drunk:

*"Oh MY GOD, listen to this crap...The initial taste is closed, opening up slowly to rich flavors of tar and chocolate, with a nose of violets."*

I was hurt when I first found out that they used to say of us "They come from another planet; thank God they found each other!" But deep down, I was proud that were not your typical Staten Island couple.

We also delighted in dairy. We adored cheeses, and we did our best to get the best. We believed for health reasons that raw milk or goats' cheeses were the choicest cheeses, and we worked hard to find raw cheeses like the ones enjoyed in Europe. The Europeans of Holland, France and Italy seemed so much healthier and oh-so sophisticated. Like my grandparents, we ate imported cheeses with impunity, especially the "Mozzarella di Bufala" (Buffalo Mozzarella) that had its own special story:

*My friends decided to get married in Italy. Upon return, they came to visit me and Cliff in Staten Island (before my family moved to Manhattan). And they told us this amazing and wonderful story about risking life and limb on a tiny moped to get to the top of a mountain in a small Italian village to get the singular and amazing taste of mozzarella made from buffalo milk. So delicious that it was well worth risking life and limb for. I risked a little less life and limb when I went to my refrigerator to take out the amazing and singular Mozzarella di Bufala that was flown in every Thursday to Chambers Street in Tribeca... literally about a block from their apartment.*

They were philosophical in seeing me revel in my revelation, and in that moment we all realized just how the world was getting so small that even the most far flung food was now available in the neighborhood.

*\*\*\**

## Recipe for Buffalo Mozzarella Salad

Here is my recipe for buffalo mozzarella salad:

- 4 large tomatoes (1.5lb).
- ½lb of fresh mozzarella (preferably buffalo).
- 1 tablespoon of olive oil.
- ½ cup of fresh basil.
- Sea salt & pepper to taste.

Alternate slices of tomatoes with slices of the cheese. Drizzle olive oil, salt and pepper, and chopped fresh basil.

An updated healthier version that my family loves adds avocado and mango, skips the cheese, and reduces or eliminates the amount of tomato (nightshade). Modify the dressing by adding some balsamic vinegar, squeezed lime juice and a teaspoon of maple syrup.

*\*\*\**

## The Milk of Human Kindness, plus Planting and Picking of Produce

We had become (relative) health food fanatics ever since we learned about Cliff's and then Jessy's serious health problems. We had started to buy some small amounts of food from health food stores, albeit reluctantly. We had given up cow's milk years ago, and switched to soy milk which we described as "chocolate milk" to our daughter Jessy. Remember those *food tricks* I told you about earlier?

Jessy thought she was so lucky to be drinking chocolate milk, until the day she came home and said,

*"Oh Mommy, you have got to buy the chocolate milk Aunt Patti buys. It tastes so much better than our chocolate milk!"*

Yes, Aunt Patti's chocolate milk was *real milk* flavored with *real chocolate.*

But real chocolate milk might contain traces of the antibiotics that were pumped into cows in order to keep them healthy in their otherwise unhealthy living conditions. In order to reduce Jessy's exposure (and possible resistance) to unnecessary antibiotics, I had doubled up my commitment to purchase only organic outdoor-reared grass-fed animal products.

As New York City dwellers, my kids never knew the joy of planting or picking vegetables that I knew as a child. But we did have the next best thing—we were often blessed with the opportunity to buy fresh food from farmers markets at nearby Union Square. Shopping turned into a fun-filled adventure; filled with songs about (in particular) all the apple varieties we came to know and love. Here's a taster of Jessy's favorite farmer's market song:

*"I love jonagold... jonnna, jonnna, jonnagold apples; I love jonagold and jonagold make me happy!"*

It might not have been good enough to win a Grammy, but it got us eating good food.

## Epigenetics and Hereditary Health: Similar, but Not the Same

While I felt fit and healthy most of the time, I was becoming a little too "hearty" (as in obese). I was flippant about being fat, and often made bad jokes about it.

*"If I get hit by a car, please eat me. I would make great road kill—mostly organic, with some nice marbling."*

I realize now that I was descending into the same disease trap that my grandparents had fallen into. My hands would swell and stiffen (like Grandma Rose), my feet would hurt (like Grandma Dorothy), and I even once woke up with a large sore red big toe (like Grandpa Nick). Maybe this was genetics at work, and I was simply doomed to inherit their illnesses. But I was younger than my grandparents were when they exhibited the same symptoms.

I had never heard of epigenetics: our ability to completely recast our genes by revisiting our food and our lifestyle. We now know that genes are like switches or the keys of a piano. Some key combinations (of food and lifestyle) produce harmonious melodies whereas others cause chaos, discordance and disease. Not only had I inherited my grandparents' genes; I had also inherited their lifestyles… with only modest adaptations, and not all of them good. I was eating much the same food as my grandparents, but in a much different place (the city) while barely moving my body. So the tune I was playing was similar… but not the same, and to my dismay not better.

# 4 – A Dark Decade of Disease and Disaster

*"That which does not kill us makes us stronger" – Nietzsche*

While you may find a few incidental foodie facts in this chapter, my main aim here is to provide a detailed account of the *decade of disease and disaster* that caused me to descend onto an unlikely path towards transformation that would ultimately lead me to reevaluate my deadly diet and lifestyle. It's a slight detour, but a worthy one.

## 21st Century Traumas

Year after traumatic year I would look at my husband and say, "Honey, we are having a bad year". Finally around the year 2008 he said, "Honey, we are having a bad decade." He was right.

In 1990, Time Magazine featured the top ten designs of the decade, including only two neighborhoods: Battery Park City (my primary home at the tip of lower Manhattan) and Seaside, Florida (my new second home). I was proud but grateful, and humbled to be an unlikely player in both of these acclaimed locations. I was also pregnant with my daughter Rose, and felt happily hormonal. My eldest daughter Jessy was four, and Cliff and I were certain it was a perfect time to expand our loving little family.

We had been living in Battery Park City for three years, and had decided to make this new neighborhood – which had been carefully planned and crafted originally on landfill from the excavation of the World Trade Center – our permanent home. The neighborhood amenities were extraordinary. The planted public areas were gorgeously extravagant, impressively tended without chemicals, and carefully overseen by Tessa Huxley (Aldous Huxley's granddaughter). The handsome residential masonry buildings were well designed, even if the apartments were tiny and unimaginative. But the primary attractions were the sweet-smelling ocean air and majestic visual beauty of New York Harbor complete with the views of Ellis Island and the Statue of

Liberty. These historic symbols never failed to evoke a sense of emotion and pride in my country and in our immigrant history.

I had felt guilty taking Jessy from our family home on Staten Island, where she had a backyard to play in, and moving her to an apartment building in lower Manhattan. I got over that quickly, when – on our first neighborhood walk on the Battery Park City promenade – she exclaimed with enthusiasm,

*"This is the BEST backyard in the whole world!"*

There was a great public school nearby in Tribeca, the expansion of which (unbeknownst to me at the time) would become a future five-year project of mine.

It was a busy time for me in Seaside, the extraordinary town that I had stumbled upon during my search for unique places to take my retired grandparents Dorothy and Carmine when I visited them in Florida. I was busy building with the brilliant architects who were designing our home there. Each night I would go to bed studying the blueprints for the house, and would fall asleep with the prints draped over me. My husband would joke about how my slowing swelling belly kept raising the blueprints higher and higher above the bed night by night. I would joke back that it was so much easier to build a baby then build a house. Designing the house was a fun, exciting time, and I looked forward to having this beautiful beach home on the Emerald Coast for my family to enjoy! The area is known not only for the unlikely emerald-colored water on Gulf of Mexico, but also the pristine white sand that Jessy would insist was snow when we first visited in the winter time… until she got out of the car to touch it.

## Dealing with Diseases

I was taking good care of myself and looking forward to the birth of our second child with great excitement. I had no particular problems during my pregnancy other than the typical trips to the bathroom. I began to notice how often my husband was taking the same trips throughout the night, so one night I asked,

*"How many times do you make this bathroom run?"*

When he reported that it was three times a night, I got really worried, because I had seen on TV how frequent  trips to the toilet could be a sign of prostate cancer. The urologist who was recommended to us discovered a large and very old urinary stricture that was preventing Cliff's bladder from emptying properly. His proposed quick fix of "rotor rooter" surgery (which had an 80 percent success rate) turned out to be a short term solution when the scar tissue came back with a vengeance and resulted in a complete urinary tract shut down. Furious that my husband now needed a urostomy – a urinary bag strapped to his leg that his bladder would empty directly into – I recall yelling at the doctor,

*"How did my young handsome husband manage to get hit by a bus in your operating room?"*

Cliff's health was impaired for many years, and he endured many surgeries. The urostomy tube puncturing the abdominal wall into his bladder had to be replaced every six weeks, which he likened to a keg of beer being tapped, and for which he was given antibiotics after each procedure. Accidents came with this condition—including the leaking of the urinary bag in an airplane and while making love (not at the same time). My youngest daughter Rose told me, when she was four, how wonderful it was to be a girl because "boys have to pee in a bag." We realized that during her entire four years of life, my husband had only every urinated into a bag.

Cliff developed candida during this time, which he fought for many months with herbs. The Alexander therapist who was helping to improve his posture recommended he see an acupuncturist. Cliff got very clever about his diet, which constituted our first major dietary reevaluation. He became a vegetarian for six months but discovered that a diet without any meat was not good for him.

All the while I was noticing that Jessy's diagnosed asthma was getting worse and worse. We tried everything: a Chinese doctor, a chiropractor, and a homeopath who blamed Jessy's lack of responsive to the homeopathic remedies on my not giving Jessy her medicine! After searching the city for someone who could figure it out, we were finally told by a doctor the horrific news that Jessy had a mutation of cystic fibrosis: a genetic disease that created lung and pancreatic disorders. The quality and ultimately the quantity of her life was to become seriously compromised.

Ironically, we learned this very bad news in the very same week that Cliff had returned from his miraculous life-changing urinary tract operation in San Francisco. It was also the same night our now-built home in Seaside, Florida got hit with a "Category 4" hurricane. I did not even bother to call the real estate managers to discover what had happened to our home that night, and I couldn't care less when I heard the good news that our house had suffered no significant damage.

*"Oh, that is nice."*

When we learned about Jessy's illness, Cliff and I were so shattered, shocked and numbed that we showed no emotion when the doctor said,

*"Do you UNDERSTAND what I am saying? Do you understand that this is serious? That you will be responsible for therapy each and every day, and that her very life is at stake?"*

We also didn't want to show the true depth of our despair in front of Jessy, who was with us at the time.

The doctor told us that she also had some good news—Jessy had no allergies, which was unusual and would make life easier for her.

*"Am I allergic to cats?"*

*"No."*

*"Great, Mommy and Daddy, can we get a cat?"*

I was allergic to cats, and I had hitherto hated them. But now I loved them.

*"That is a great idea Jessy, yes of course we can get some cats."*

In fact, we would have agreed to a horse or anything to make her happy.

Of course, we had no idea what the therapy would be like. It was dreadful. Our kitchen was taken over by nebulizers that had to be sterilized over and over for multiple medicines. The manual therapy consisted of systematic pounding on Jessy's tiny body to make her cough-cough-cough, spit-spit-spit. A few hours later, it was time to do it again. Since my husband was recovering from a serious surgery, he could not really help. I was delirious, exhausted, and terrified that I was neglecting our lovely youngest child Rose.

Jessy was furious with all the therapy and medicines she was subjected to. She tortured me, and when I begged her to be kinder to me she said,

*"Mommy, if I do not take out my anger on you, I will take it out on my friends... and they are just little girls."*

I had to agree that I was a better candidate.

Not merely difficult, this was the first of our "surreal" years. It was so surreal to see Jessy surrounded by her lovely friends on her 10<sup>th</sup> birthday, all singing the birthday song (in different languages), and with me wondering how many more birthdays she would actually have.

Could I ever be happy again? One of her doctors, who also had the disease, said,

*"You will never be happy that your daughter has cystic fibrosis, but you will be happy again."*

It took about a year for us to adjust to the challenging new normal. We made a secret pact to treat Jessy no different to how we did before the diagnosis, and to never ever to feel sorry for her; to continue to live our lives as best we could, including the continuation of my businesses, community responsibilities, and the projects that made me proud:

*I was building another new building in Seaside, Florida, and was establishing a new business there.*

*I was a community leader in lower Manhattan where I had a law practice.*

*I was the president of my condominium building of 500 units in Battery Park City.*

*I was getting unhealthy!*

## Diet Dilemmas

Our diet remained an issue of constant concern and consideration, and the Cystic Fibrosis (CF) organization presented us with a diet dilemma by encouraging us to "fatten" Jessy with fast food and canned chemical-laced products even though she was a perfect weight for her height. We figured for ourselves a clear connection between milk and mucus, despite the CF society mandating milk and other dairy products.

We were ridiculed by parents and doctors alike for our forthright views about other ways to bulk up our daughter with nuts, avocados and seeds rather than ice cream sundaes. We were also ridiculed for our insistence that dark leafy greens could compete with cream in terms of calcium content. The doctors thought that Jessy was doomed to a life with brittle bones, and yet...

*She tested to have the strongest bones of any kid her age!*

Our devotion to her whole food diet and physical therapy seemed to pay off wonderfully. She never went to the hospital and never got very sick.

## A Beautiful Day Gone Very Bad

September 11, 2001 was a beautiful day about to go bad. Far beyond bad!

Our life in Battery Park City had evolved. I was in a brand new apartment in a brand new building above the school that my daughter Rose had just started in the 6th grade. I felt a great sense of pride at having been a primary "player" in development of this complex community project that was built on budget and on time.

On that morning, I woke up in the arms of my handsome husband. I lingered a long while after our early alarm call, and we made love for as long as we dared before the arrival of my 7am taxi. The taxi was due to take me to a photo shoot for my acclaimed Florida art supply and toy store business in Seaside, Florida where my staff was taking me out for my birthday. As I got out of bed, I heard and enjoyed the sounds of children outside my window. The children sounded intensely happy, playing in the new ball field that I had helped usher in as the Battery Park City Chairperson.

Suddenly I did not want to leave my family. My two angelic daughters were still sleeping soundly in the other bedroom when something suddenly came over me. I went back to bed with my husband who was sleepy and dreamy from the lovemaking.

*"We have to stay connected"*

*"Of course, sweetheart, I will call you."*

*"No, no. I mean here." (pointing to my heart, then his)*

*"Yes, of course."*

I knew the tone. He was humoring me, as kindly as he could.

Now I had to rush to shower and dress before the taxi turned up. Which of course it did before I was dressed. I entered the elevator without kissing my daughters goodbye, and resolved to call them as soon as I got to the airport and before they left for school.

After settling into the back seat, and as the taxi made its way up the West Side Highway, I looked out the back window to see my neighborhood looking so beautiful. The light was clear and bright. The temperature was perfect. It was a perfect day. Not for the first time this morning, suddenly something felt terribly wrong. I wanted to *go back*, not merely *look back*.

Our apartment was only half a block away from the World Trade Center, which provided the view from every one of our apartment windows. When the attack happened, Rose and Cliff were at the foot of the World Trade Center— Cliff in our apartment, and Rose in her brand new classroom. Jessy had gone to her high school (the Professional Performing Arts School) which was uptown and completely isolated. I was sitting in Newark airport with a close clear view of lower Manhattan when the horror unfolded at what would henceforth be forever known as "ground zero".

## Two Towers of Terror

I experienced a jolt that could never be forgotten, and I knew that in that moment the world had changed forever. One minute I was trying to decide where to go for my birthday dinner with my staff in Seaside, Florida, and the next minute I saw smoke. There had been some kind of accident, apparently at the top of the World Trade Tower. My plane was being called for boarding. Should I stay or should I go? We had lived through the first bombing of the World Trade Center in 1993, but I would soon learn this was different. I watched one tower fall... then (sometime later) the other one. The debris looked like it covered the whole of lower Manhattan. When my cell phone would not work, I headed for the payphone. It rang and rang... but no answer.

With the phones still not working and the airport news blacked out, in my shocked state I began plotting all kinds of crazy ideas. I could find a boat to take me back to lower Manhattan to find Rose. If Rose and Cliff were dead (God forbid!) I calmly calculated that I could still get to Manhattan and find Jessy, who would surely know what was happening... but not what to do.

I was getting my news from a nearby bar. When the second tower tumbled, the commentator had said,

*"Well, the last report stated that the children 'were' safe... but I do not know now. The school is much closer to the second tower."*

I realized that it was not only about *my child* and *my husband*. I had potentially just witnessed the deaths of hundreds, thousands, or even tens of thousands of people. I was screaming,

*"All those people! All those people! All those souls!"*

To my great relief, and via a convoluted communication loop that involved the staff of my Seaside stores, I discovered that Cliff and Rose had not been killed and were wandering around Manhattan. Alive, at least.

But what about Jessy? I saw smoke, an insane amount of smoke that wasn't at all friendly to Jessy's cystic fibrosis. Could my staff contact her too via her school?

The Hotel and the "No Tell" Motel

In the meantime the airport was bedlam. Thousands of us were suddenly stranded and the police had no idea about what to do or where to send people. I insanely stood directly in front of a Holiday

Inn bus to force it to stop, not caring at all if the bus crashed into me. The driver seemed oblivious to unfolding events as he actually asked me if I had a reservation for the Holiday Inn.

*"Sure I do, and so do all these other people."*

While we could get to the hotel, it became obvious that no one would be getting into Manhattan any time soon. I used the hotel phone to call my frantic Dad in Pennsylvania, who told me to take the train or bus *away from the city* (and away from what we now knew to be a terrorist attack) so that he could pick me up without becoming hopelessly mired in the web of the city traffic chaos. After a few confused messages via my staff in Florida, Cliff was now disconnected from me, which made my earlier premonition (that we should "stay connected") all the more prescient. Against the odds, he and Rose did eventually find Jessy, and he decided to take them all to Staten Island to be with family. Not the safest plan, I thought, since they would have to travel past the two towers – or what was left of them – again. All that smoke on poor Jessy's lungs!

The Holiday Inn was too booked-up for the bus full of unexpected guests, so the staff encouraged us all to look for motel rooms before they all got booked up too. I went on a gypsy cab journey to find the first motel with available rooms, which was more "no tell" (sleazy, with mirrored ceilings in the rooms) than motel. I cried, and cried, and it wasn't pretty. As my husband has told me—I'm not one of those women who inexplicably look terrific when in tears.

The telephone in my room did not work, so I huddled in the lobby with a big-hearted black bus driver who accompanied me in heartfelt prayer to hear from my family. I did one of those "God deals"—that I would never ever ask for anything ever again if our Dearest Lord kept my family alive. Our prayers were answered at 7pm when the motel phone rang with news from my dear sister Patti Ann who confirmed that Cliff, Jessy and Rose had indeed made it to Staten Island. It was eleven hours after the first attack, and the longest eleven hours of my life. I now knew about Cliff and my girls, but not my cats... who I had forgotten to include in my "God deal". A deal was a deal, and I remained steadfast that it was too late for me to pray for the cats now, so the big friendly bus driver began to solemnly pray for them on my behalf.

And so began the long wait for someone to pick me up for the journey into New Jersey that would be defined by even more drama. Cliff and my brother Jeffery collected me the next afternoon. I already knew how it felt to be "alone in a crowd," but I never expected to feel alone in the presence of the two people (apart from my children) that I loved the most. I was definitely disconnected, and actually angry that Cliff had not gone straight to Jessy and then straight to a hotel. But he was in shock. I was in shock. We all were in shock. It took days before I could feel much of *anything* again.

My friend Ruth was in Europe, but managed to get us the keys to her studio apartment in the Upper West Side of Manhattan. Those next few days there were some of the happiest days of my life.

*"I love you, Mommy."*

*"I love you, Jessy."*

*"I love you, Daddy."*

*"I love you, Jessy."*

*"I love you, Rose."*

*"I love you Mommy."*

*"I love you Daddy."*

*"I love you Rose."*

As our hearts healed, our humor returned. Cliff continued this lovefest with "I love you John-boy" as an amusing allusion to the TV show The Waltons. For a few precious days, we were together morning (and mourning), noon and night in a studio apartment. All I could think about was love, gratitude… and *food*. With my American Express card, we began eating our way up Columbus Avenue restaurant-by-restaurant. We acted like we were on vacation, and it seemed so strange that the uptown people were so able to dismiss the fires downtown. We were alive and we were happy, and I thought I would be happy forever because we had witnessed the worst and made it through. Surely life had nothing left to throw at us. But sadly, there would soon be yet another test. When taking the children to Rose's temporary school, we heard the announcement of the anthrax attacks in the ABC building next door to Ruth's apartment building.

## Collecting the Cats, and Moving On

When we finally collected our cats – who had chewed on every cable and cord in the apartment – we saw that the fires from the towers were still nowhere near being put out. The air was filled with a terrible acrid-metallic smell, and although the authorities told us we could move back home in just a few weeks' time, our noses told us a different story. We would have to find another place to live… possibly permanently.

One day we were allowed to walk into Battery Park City from Canal Street so as to collect some of our belongings. We took the trek with shopping carts, through the succession of stops and identity verification checks defining a newly-established police state that now replaced our previously perceived paradise. Upon reaching the 24th floor of our building – step by exhausting step – we saw how the previous enviable views from the windows of our apartment building had now been replaced by scenes of utter devastation. A grand apocalypse of still-burning buildings (or what was left of them). A vision of hell, with streams of smoke coming seemingly from the very bowels of the earth. We couldn't breathe; it broke our hearts. And our hearts broke some more when we heard the torrent of answer machine messages that were testament of the sad day's events: me hoping that Cliff was still in the apartment and could search for Rose at school; Jessy begging to know what to do, and getting more and more manic as time ticked on. We packed what we could, mostly Jessy's therapy machines and medicines, and decided to ditch the rest. Then we wended our way back uptown in a long line of dismal people, each one wondering what would become of their newly disrupted lives.

The trail of tears brought us into the smoke-filled Tribeca, where the famished Cliff decided to try and find a restaurant. Like an oasis in the desert, we did manage to find an open café that turned out not to be a mere mirage. We tried to fit our bulky belongings as best we could next to a lovely table, and we ordered a goat cheese salad with two glasses of chardonnay as though it was "business as usual." The food was delicious and comforting, and we quickly began to count our many blessings. While our previously very privileged lives had been turned upside-down, it still did not compare with the true hardships that many people face in the world each and every day. "Food for thought" indeed.

We decided to flee New York in favor of our second home and toy / art store business in the pure paradise of panhandle Florida. I could not plan our escape fast enough—Cliff and Jessy would drive with our cats in the back seat of our car, and I would fly down to Florida with Rose. The plan was perfect, even though we still had the problem of finding new work and new schools for our children. And first, we had planned to celebrate Jessy's 16th birthday.

We did not want to deprive Jessy of her special day on October 1, 2001. She wanted to see all of her friends and family before we left the city, so we hosted the birthday party on a beautiful ship that sailed around lower Manhattan. What seemed like the perfect plan just a few weeks before, now seemed bizarre, even cruel. I was so worried that her birthday would be spoiled as we sailed past our burning neighborhood, that I had contacted the ship to see if we could avoid the burning embers of the two towers. But the route was pre-approved and could not be changed.

Arguably the best birthday present for Jessy, who was an aspiring actress by now, was the national rollout (on the day of her birthday) of the first commercial she had filmed. My daughter became the "Paxil" girl when everyone in the entire world seemed to need the anti-depression medication; the anti-depression medication that had originally been due to be advertised on 9/11 (but which the advertiser thought it would be too unseemly). Even as I cried throughout the party, Jessy and her performer pals demonstrated how "the show must go on" by dancing on the tables and chairs.

With a hired driver and truck I was able to muscle through the multitudes of homeland security to reach our old apartment; to recover our furniture and have it delivered to Staten Island. While securing our property back on Staten Island, we bumped into Cliff's first cousin who told us that her brother Paul – a firefighter with a wife and two children – had been killed in the tower attack. No one had told us this, or the fact that his aunt had suffered a heart attack upon hearing the news, because the family felt we had enough to deal with. This very personal and very permanent news hit us hard. This was family. And this was death.

A few days before we left, I was bringing the girls to their makeshift school. I wanted my kids out of NYC. Now I started to get really angry, and began to rant.

*"I hate this. I hate them. Those f****in' terrorists do not know who they are dealing with. We will find them. We will crush them. We will kill every last one of the...."*

*"There is a Republican as President. They are ruthless. GOOD!! Mark my words, I said. We will get these bastards in a week, maybe two tops."*

My little girls stared up at me. Jessy with her blonde hair and blue eyes and heart shaped face. Rose with her pale skin and pink cheeks, light brown hair and wide open green eyes. Both looking like angels standing in the gateway of hell with the fire and smoke in the back ground. They spoke—

*"Mommy. You know that hate makes more hate, Mommy. You know that, Mommy. Hate just makes more hate."*

I will never love those kids more than at that moment.

## Death of a Dear Friend

As per our plan, Cliff and Jessy would drive and I would fly down to Florida with Rose. So we left for Seaside a few days later.

Rose and I were met from the plane by my best friend and manager of our toy and art supply store—Quincy's. Lloyd Ann was a warm wise woman. I loved her. My staff and customers all loved her. Her family adored her. She sprinted like an eleven-year-old right past Rose and me (sitting on a bench) and right into the airport, waiving a handful of tiny American flags left over from our 4th of July festivities the summer before. And she had gotten Rose her "uniform" tee shirts for the Seaside Charter School that would be her temporary school. We were weary and war-torn, but relieved to be there in Seaside… our escape from hell.

Next morning, the phone rang. Lloyd Ann was gone. Her son Milam delivered the unexpected news that she had gone home, fallen to the floor with barely a thud, and been found dead by her husband Jim. That was it.

Rose was running around the house trying to close all the windows to shut in the deafening screams. My screams. Although I continued to scream, I could not feel much of anything. Yet even with so much recent destruction and death, including Cliff's firefighter first cousin, I was more profoundly affected with this single passing of a woman I had loved so dearly. The staff and I all were solemn when we closed down the store and watched as friends and customers began placing bunches of flowers once the news got out in town. The passing of Lloyd Ann was so life-shattering for so many that I feel embarrassed to make it part of "my" story. But it is part of my story. I couldn't believe that I had lost a key colleague and dear friend.

Lloyd Ann's husband Jim also worked for me, and was pitifully shattered. He said over and over,

*"I do not remember the last I time I told her that I loved her. Promise me Dorothy… that you will tell the people you love that you love them. Say it often, because you never know when something like this could happen. Promise me."*

Life was just life, and would remain a mystery. Love was the only force that could steady you for the ride. When Cliff and Jessy finally arrived I wanted to bring us all into Quincy's art class room and "crazy glue" us all together.

## Movie Set, Dream World, or Nightmare Scenario?

Seaside was the town where Jim Carey's movie The Truman Show had been filmed a few years earlier, at exactly the same time that our building was being built, so our house had to be digitally deleted from many scenes. Jessy had even been filmed for the movie, but unfortunately didn't make it into the final cut. In the movie, Truman is the unwitting stooge in a soap opera filmed for audience entertainment, with the twist being that he actually thinks he's living his very own ordinary life. I began to wonder whether life was imitating art; whether my own life – and its improbable events – was really my own. Was I on a movie set, or in a lucid dream from which I would soon awake?

We lost a lot in 9/11. My law practice had been located near to ground zero, and I had foolishly accepted a large loan to rebuild it, but there was no business to build back up. We used the money to live while we waited for things to return to normal. But years after the fires went out, there was no return to normal. Each disaster that momentarily fills the TV screens fades from view as soon as the next one comes along somewhere in the world. But the survivors struggle on out of sight. I remember a bill collector hammering me one day in 2004, three years after the event. I told him I had not yet recovered from 9/11, to which he replied,

*"Seriously. I mean, that is so over. Take some responsibility."*

I had taken responsibility in my life. I was a passionate mother of a child with a serious disease, who had to follow a punishing protocol to keep her healthy. I owned two businesses and had staff. I had been a community leader. I had developed a strategy to build a school for the children in the community. And more. I knew responsibility, and had worked hard for my community, family and clients. Over-worked and way-over-stressed, but disasters do not discriminate between those who can cope and those who can't.

My businesses were wholly dependent on me and the people I could attract, and they began to fall apart. The families and small businesses that I served were gone, and those that remained needed charity as they struggled to survive. The disaster loan was secured against my home in Florida, and with Manhattan looking so messy we decided to expand our business in the south.

The expansion of our toy store was a disaster of my own devising. I had been courted by a "big wig" in Alabama and one of my dearest friends who I loved. She was a gorgeous talented woman who made every moment memorable, and she promised she would help me. With nothing working out in New York, and with the Florida business too small to support us, this opportunity out of nothing seemed like a gift from God. Maybe too good to be true.

I knew nothing about Birmingham, Alabama. But I did have a best friend from there, and I knew at least ten awesome and very cool people who lived there and loved our Seaside store. They would come to our art classes, they seemed to appreciate my love for sensual fine art supplies and old world toys, and we would party with them all of the time. I cooked for them all, and they loved my food. Charles, a food magazine photographer, claimed that he worked with chefs from all over the world, but I was the "real deal" home cook.

We built a beautiful store in Birmingham; amazing, and acclaimed by all of the press. But our hip, happening, urban storefront did not last a single year in this "shopping mall" town. The new business in Birmingham imploded, taking our savings (and those of our loved-ones) with it. This was this last straw that nearly broke *me*, let alone the proverbial camel's back. When I left an attorney's office and started to pee in the streets of lower Manhattan, it was finally time to start piling on the pills.

When not peeing in the streets, I was suffering from an accompanying irritable bowel syndrome, but didn't entirely lose my sense of humor. I called my investor friends who helped themselves to some merchandise ("the menopause bandits") but I couldn't be mad at them despite everything I had done to make the project a success—including taking out a huge second mortgage on my much-beloved Florida home. I had intended to die there, but not at age 48.

## Winds of Change

The *winds of change* had made things even worse, and we had to leave Battery Park City which we had tried gallantly to re-inhabit to "show" those terrorists that they could not break us New Yorkers. But once again, they sure showed us. The neighborhood we knew on September 10th, 2001 no longer existed. It was still a mess, and (we discovered) absurdly toxic. Our new home base became my childhood home on Staten Island where I was raised, and this would be the base from which we would try to rebuild our lives. Rose was enrolled in Manhattan's prestigious Beacon High School, and did her best to stay with friends in Manhattan whenever she could. I spent most of my time in Florida, where I had sold the house but kept a lease for the store.

Due to the *winds of technological change*, I figured that the internet was the future for a small store wanting to sell to the world. So I decided to grow the internet side of the store that had been featured in many national magazines including Time Magazine. It seemed smart, but it was not. Although Amazon was mostly just selling books on the internet, it was about to dominate other areas of online retail sales, and I could not compete.

I believe in hard work, and I was ready to work as hard as necessary to pay back (with interest) all those who had invested in my initiatives. And to give back the future that I had once given to (and had to take back from) my children. But the *winds of change* blew again, quite literally.

I could write that the "unimaginable" happened again, but in the Gulf of Mexico hurricanes are quite imaginable. In Seaside there is one huge season called summer. All of the money for the year is earned in 12 weeks, and then the hurricanes come. But in 2005 they came early.

The summer of 2005 was the summer of the famous Hurricane Katrina. But our town of Seaside had already seen its share of huge storms, so we prepared to simply sit it out. In the air after the storm were tiny beautiful bits of froth from the ocean water. These "flowers" (which we thought they were at first) were so delicate and pretty, oxymoronic in front of the furious dark and deafening water. I knew I would do anything to prevent closing the business and firing my loving and loyal terrified staff, but I also knew that all might soon be lost. I remained completely calm while contemplating what lay ahead—the unending pitiless pull from the creditors; robbing Peter to pay Paul, but doing no real business at all. Ever the optimist, I took out more loans until the latest wind of change blew over.

Bill Clinton is quoted as once saying during a presidential campaign,

*"It's the economy, stupid."*

And now it really was. First the economy of Florida, and then the economy of the entire United States careened towards collapse. Just like natural disasters, financial depressions don't discriminate between those who are safely solvent and those who are already "depressed."

## PTSD, Pity and Pills

More and more, I was finding comfort in food—graduating from glasses of wine to whole bottles, and eating cheese like it was mother's milk (not to mention the bread and pasta). I craved meat, and I remember running into Seaside's Modica Market and screaming like a banshee for Charlie Modica to cut me up a hunk of "dead animal."

Post-Traumatic Stress Disorder (PTSD). I did not think I had it. I did not seek counseling. I regarded myself as "ordinarily" stressed, and merely popped the pills that the doctor prescribed. Even my family seemed to think I was fine, but it wasn't fine to be living my life through a lens of thick dense fog. There was nothing "ambient" about my Ambien, and the sleeping pills weren't helping me sleep at all.

There's a fine line between genius and madness, and one of our greatest ever geniuses had this to say about insanity:

*"It's doing the same thing over and over, and expecting a different result."*

Which was exactly what I was doing. My decisions made no sense, and my risks got riskier. My anxiety was agonizing and my depression was debilitating.

Maybe *doing something different* would yield a different result, but I would have laughed out loud at anyone who had dared suggest that diet and lifestyle changes could make all the difference. I mean—you don't run out with a cup of herbal tea to someone who was just hit by a bus!

But maybe…

# 5 – Prescription Pills and the Transformation Train

*"It ain't what you don't know that gets you into trouble. It's what you know for sure that just ain't so." – Mark Twain*

In 2011 I realized that my doctor had absolutely no idea how to help me. He too realized he could not help me, because he was trained to find and treat disease symptoms rather than the root causes of those diseases. His statement to me was quite clear and direct—"YOU have to do something about your health."

The doctor's waiting room was brimming with people as diseased and obese as I was. And so were the offices, schools and supermarkets that I visited. Clearly, I was part of an epidemic. Since there were no simple solutions offered by the conventional health care system, those solutions would have to be sought in the alternative healing and self-care systems, but this too would not be so simple. If healing was easy, why were there so many people still standing in the same unhealthy shoes as me? There were some serious problems to solve. I was morbidly obese, with irritable bowel syndrome and diverticulitis. I suffered from depression, anxiety and insomnia and was addicted to the pills that controlled those conditions. My triglycerides were at 230. I found it difficult to walk, and my children had to "tow" me around the block.

## What's the Alternative?

When it came to healing my family, I had always used food and alternative medicine to complement the traditional health care system, with the result that my family was healthy while I was not. Having spent a lifetime studying and cooking apparently-healthy food, I remained adamant that I had at least a 90% healthy diet and that I was still salvageable… if we conveniently forget that dying young thing! I was nothing if not confident that (to paraphrase the X-Files) "the truth was out there," and that I would find the true road to healthy redemption via the wonder of the World Wide Web. One way or another I would find the illusive diet, pill, potion or procedure that would get me thin and healthy in no time at all.

I began my research into diets with great determination and dedication. I Googled away and read everything I could. I searched all the best and most popular self-health books on Amazon.

*Within weeks I was more confused than ever.*

The extraordinary amount of information on the internet was confusing and often contradictory. Too much noise, and not enough signal. Eat this but not that. Eat grains but no meat (vegetarian). Eat meat but no grains (paleo or Atkins). Walk but don't run. Run but don't walk. Yoga is good for anxiety… but will make you fat. I began to panic that I did not have a plan; that my 12-hour work days did not afford sufficient time for me to figure it all out. It became clear that after all my years of healthy eating advocacy, I still had no idea how to determine the best diet for me. Well, not one that would yield permanent results rather than the short-term fixes of my prior fad diets that were usually not even short-term fixes at all because they often caused me to *gain even more weight back*.

## Health Help at Hand

It became increasingly clear that I needed some expert health advice, so I decided to reach out to the best and most trusted alternative health care experts I knew. I remembered that Dr. Cliff Inkles had given me a referral for a health coach several years earlier when I was working with him after 9/11. I adored and admired Dr. Cliff, so – while still unsure about what a health coach could do for me – I set out to find her card. Despite several home moves, and the fact I never find anything without turning the whole house upside down, I found her card in just five minutes. A good omen. The "Path for Life" card directed me to a very attractive web site with an article that included a photograph of an artichoke. The artichoke is my favorite vegetable (another good omen) and I use an artichoke for my own logo today.

I called Jeanette immediately and made an appointment. I really did not know what a "health coach" was exactly, but I knew that I needed one. Danish health coach Jeanette Bronée turned out to be the very attractive, intelligent, and cool health coach who I had faith  would save me.

My first objective was to eliminate prescription drugs, which I believed were the cause of my liver's unhealthy enzymes. Since my doctor had forced me off of Ambien (which I had grown to love), I honestly thought he would encourage me to get off the Effexer and Clonozapan too. But his PA, Keith, told me it was probably too late. Nonetheless, I persuaded him to put me on a protocol to get off the pills in a week or two. He had no faith that I would succeed, but I had all the faith I needed. And I sure needed it. I fully expected to be uncomfortable. I expected to be sad, and I expected to be sick—even very sick. But a few days into the withdrawal protocol I got seriously sick. I thought I would die. Seriously, DIE.

*I did not expect to have brain zaps.*

Over and over and over, ZAP-ZAP-ZAP. It felt like I was getting electrocuted. Gently electrocuted, but electrocuted all the same. These zaps were not nearly as painful as they were scary, which was ironic because I was getting off the depression and anxiety medications for the very reason that they had made me feel terrified. Now the withdrawal symptoms were terrifying me too. I could not work. I could not sleep.

I understood why Keith thought I could not come off the pills. I called him, and begged him to offer me anything for temporary respite from these horrific symptoms. He said he was concerned about compounding the problem with additional drugs, and suggested we slow down or backtrack on the withdrawal protocol. But I did not want to go *back*; I wanted to go *forward*.

## Getting My Brain Back

Enter the internet, which turned out to be a lifesaver in this instance. I found others who had the brain zaps, and found assurance that they would stop.

Then it hit me. How the heck were those pills affecting my brain if this is how I felt when I came off them? I had this crazy idea that these pills had been innocuous, that they were just "naturally" recirculating or re-uptaking the existing very *natural* serotonin within my brain. I thought that this new strategy to "cure" depression was amazing, and that it sounded almost healthy. But I also knew how bad I felt when I forgot to take a pill and it was like the plug was being pulled out of my very being; like the world was coming to an end. The upshot to this is that the terrible withdrawal symptoms actually encouraged me to stick with the withdrawal protocol, because the mere absence of the medications demonstrated just how powerful these pills had been… and hence how important it was for my body and brain to be rid of them.

I wanted my brain back. I needed my brain back. And I was determined to get it back.

## Project of a Lifetime

Meanwhile I had a really amazing job helping people at the largest not-for-profit corporation in the coolest part of Brooklyn! I was busy buying senior citizen centers and developing all kinds of interesting and novel social service programs. I was writing grants like a mad woman, and was generally being a purposeful human being.

*I was also developing what I believed would be a project of a lifetime.*

I was developing a proposal for Medicaid-funded private health insurance companies that covered people within our homecare service programs. I was attending senior centers to help subsidize fresh vegetables and whole grains that would dramatically improve the quality and nutrition of the food they were being served… and I wanted to document the health results. I dreamt that this endeavor – reduce illness by combining better food with more exercise – would spearhead a new National Medicaid pilot program that would benefit the insurance companies without requiring additional public expenditure.

I had resurrected a significant grant of $400,000 that was almost a blank check from the State of New York for this important project. It could be the work of a lifetime, and an amazing fusion of food and law (my two passions). I was so excited that I started to feel like I might actually heal. I felt commitment, passion, and a purpose in life. I was making good money, paying down my debts, and looking forward to a bright future.

## My "Out-of-Body" Experience, and the Path to Progress

The fat body that I felt trapped inside had functioned as mere pedestal for my brain for a very long time. My brain had become disconnected from my body to the extent that my whole life was a true "out of body experience"—perhaps like the ones people get when they are near to death. Judging from the doctor's diagnosis about my potential lifespan, my life had actually become a "near death experience" too.

My health coach, Jeanette, saw me or spoke to me once a week. We started with diet, but quickly got deep into my "nourishment" needs. I wanted to get out of this body, but Jeannette wanted me to go deep into it. To be honest I was not even certain what she meant. I was also a bit afraid. If we dug too deep, I didn't know what we would find.

To be healthy, I had to live in the body that I had moved out of a long time before. I had to move back in and find a way to integrate my body back into my life. What's more, I had to do it myself. Jeanette does not tell you what to do, but merely points your own inner voice in the right direction. It was tough to take (that I would have to do all the hard work myself) but I had faith in my teacher. Why? Because Jeanette had surely suffered herself, and had come out the other side. So I was determined to progress through her "Path for Life" step-by-step until I too made it out the other side.

I developed a mantra:

*Just do the work.*

*Just do the work.*

*Just do the work.*

I started to learn about food, and to my great shock discovered that I had not been eating the best of foods for me. We worked on food first by modifying my Mediterranean diet, and I started to lose a few pounds. Then WHAAAAMMMM...

## From Fired Up to Fired, and a Friend's Funeral

I had made my usual mistake of believing that I was now firmly on the path to progress, that I had fully used up my life's quota of bad things, and that my new job had been my "reward" for making it this far. But in the blink of an eye I went from being "fired up" (about my recent achievements) to being "fired" (from my job). A corporate re-organization left the remaining managers jockeying for a safe position. I stayed out of the fray while focusing on my projects, and found myself on the outside looking in.

*I thought I'd do that job until I retired, but now I was fat, over fifty, and fired!*

What a cruel episode of my real-life Truman Show this was.

I went home despondent, to be greeted with an urgent message to call back my best friend Colleen in New Hampshire. Her husband Jack answered, and began babbling that... really... it was nothing. I figured it probably was nothing compared with the fact that I had just been fired from the job I loved, but something told me to persist until Jack came clean.

*"Oh,"* Jack said, *"It's just that I'm dying."*

*"Apparently I have pancreatic cancer and it has been working on me for a long time. They've given me two months to live."*

At Jack's funeral I tried to explain who he had been to me, and what he had meant to me. He was my favorite friend, and his wife Colleen was my best friend. He was such good company. We both loved food. We both loved family. And we loved each other even though we argued all of the time… about all the important issues like fruits and vegetables (and how to cook them). To be fair, we did also have deep discussions about life, the universe and everything—often through the night.

Being fifteen years older than us, Jack was our de facto "placeholder pal." We didn't have to think about death until he went first. So now it was time to mull over my own mortality, but my newly-off-the-pills brain and body chemistry could not take it. I went to a place I never visited before. A place of deep, deep existential fear. A place far deeper even than hell.

## Boarding the Transformation Train

For the first time in my life I understood how people felt when they contemplated committing suicide. I had always enjoyed life far too much to understand. Oh, those poor people. Poor me. It nearly drove me back to the pills, and I even drove to the doctor's office to get some. The pills that I procured sat on my counter in the kitchen, beckoning me, but at the same time stiffening my resolve not to take them. Since they were there for me to take *tomorrow* (if I really needed to), then I didn't really need to take them *today*. Then tomorrow became today, and I could always wait *just one more day*.

I have no idea how I managed to stay off of the pills, but I know I could not have done it without Jeanette. She had complete faith in me. She helped me focus on foods such as brown rice and vegetables… all washed down with green tea. She had me take walks in nature. To my astonishment, I learned about studies indicating that food and movement could be as effective as pills in treating depression. I could feel the food and movement creating a new me. Not all at once, but I had at least boarded the transformation train.

# 6 – You Are What You Eat

In my mind, food was not the issue, so in order to improve my health I simply had to deal with the residual trauma in my body resulting from my prior emotional injuries. After resolving my emotional issues and my remaining "real life" problems, my body would get healthy on its own. Or so I thought.

I thought I had already succeeded in removing all unhealthy food from my diet many years before. I had a good diet, I ate very healthy food, and I did not need to change much about the food I ordinarily ate. Just a few tweaks here and there. Or so I thought.

On some level I was convinced that my only real food issue was that I ate too much of it relative to how much I moved; which ironically is what my doctor was hinting at when he offered me that book of calorie counting. Getting slim was simply a matter of getting the input and output energy balance right, right? Eat less, and exercise more. Simple.

So it was pretty hard for me to learn the truth about the effect my food choices were having on my body.

## You Are What You Eat (and Digest)

Do you eat to live, or live to eat? I think the answer is yes to both, with some explanation. In the natural world it seems obvious that most if not all creatures (apart from humans) *eat to live*. But animals eat food perfectly suited to them and created in nature just for them. New studies indicate that they do not thrive if the food is made tasteless. They seem to both *eat to live* and *live to eat* in perfect harmony. Another fascinating new study proved that women who ate food that they did not like did not fully absorb the nutrients in the food. In my world it was quite obvious that all-too-often I was mostly *living to eat*. The food I was eating out of sheer habit was not serving me, nourishing me, supporting me, or even truly feeding me. It was *entertaining me* and *connecting me to my family heritage.* It was clearly not what nature intended for me.

I felt like the food "playing field" had been changed and the goalposts had been moved when my health coach, Jeanette, provided me with some hard-to-accept new food "knowledge". The "new rules" would *seriously* upset and challenge me. But I learned that the function of food should not be for mere entertainment, divorced from its sacred purpose of building a new me. My new food choices would be the ingredients in the recipe to cook up the new Dorothy.

## Ditching the Dairy

Milk is a perfect food for infants of the same species. Cats' milk is good for kittens and cows' milk is good for calves. But it does not follow that cats' milk is good for calves any more than cows' milk is good for kittens. Only humans drink the milk of other species, and it should come as no surprise that most of us are intolerant of it… whether we know this or not. Add into the mix what is added to the milk without your knowledge: the antibiotics that are pumped into cattle to counter the diseases they develop as a result of being fed a poor diet in the first place. Then subtract from the mix the nutrients that are killed off (along with the germs, admittedly) by the pasteurization process. Have you ever considered that no mother needs to pasteurize her own milk before feeding it to baby, does she?

Jeannette had something to say about milk and cheese; even the raw milk cheeses; and the European cheeses that I thought made the Mediterraneans ever-so healthy. She encouraged me to test how cheese affected me. And by becoming a food detective, I started to understand.

The dairy issue was all about me. I carefully monitored how I *felt* after I ate cheese, and there was no doubt—within just a few minutes after eating cheese, I could not breathe through my nose. Since I already knew that cream contributed to my irritable bowel syndrome (IBS) it should have come as no surprise at all to discover that cheese wasn't compatible with me either. And since I loved my cheese – several times per day, and particularly on pizza – it was not good news that the cheese *did not love me back*. So I set about substituting the cheese and other dairy components of my diet.

I substituted hummus, avocados, nut butters and nut "cheeses" for real cheese. I enjoyed those substitutions so much that my dairy decreased from a two-or-three-times-per-day staple to a two-or-three-times-per-month delicacy. From daily to rarely.

## Banishing the Bread (and Pasta)

I can still smell the doughy smell of the pasta drying in Grandma Rose's flour-covered kitchen. And I can't escape the Holtermann's 100-year heritage in the bakery business on Staten Island. For years we ate only the finest breads and pastas: delicious crusty whole wheat bread (especially my beloved sourdough) and only Italian imported pasta cooked al dente just as my grandparents did (and as Dr. Andrew Weill continues to recommend).

I learned a long time ago that white flour is stripped of all nutrients, so I had already moved my family onto whole wheat bread. But "I" continued to consume the *carbs* despite the 1-2 pounds of weight piling onto my body every month. I ate all the carbs I could, because I had bought into the belief that *fat* was the real enemy. What could be more logical than the assertion that *fat makes you fat?*

Jeanette had some bad news about bread and my beloved pasta. These were identified as prime suspects in the crime of making me ill. Bad news indeed, because—how could I continue to be Italian if I had to ditch the dough? Jeanette painstakingly taught me the difference between *whole grains* (that you could see as "grainy" with your own eyes) and *processed flour*. She told me it was not safe even to seek sanctuary in "whole wheat flour" unless you could see the grain.

Just as with the cheese, I set about testing how I felt after eating bread, but the result was not so clear cut this time. On the one hand, where was the harm in bread that turned out to not have the immediate negative effect that dairy did? On the other hand, I noticed that I did feel lighter and did eat more vegetables when I did away with dough. It was a true dilemma, because – while I didn't go as far as my Grandma Dorothy in feeding toast to animals – I did delight in my own coffee-and-toast mornings.

Against the odds (but obviously not against the grain) I stopped eating flour products almost entirely. I started to eat only whole grains that I could actually "see", and I equated flour with the sugar that I already knew was no good for me. Whole grains made me feel fantastic, and gave me energy for hours after I ate them. It may not have been an easy adjustment, but I was committed to change and I trusted the process of being mindful of exactly what I ate and how it affected my body and brain.

## Substitutions and Strategies

I switched to brown rice pasta, and also decided I would enjoy high quality imported pasta from Italy on special occasions because I could cook it al dente (still a bit chewy to the teeth) to lower its glycemic index. The lower the GI, the less sugar running amok in your blood and through your body. This particular pasta was a traditional strain rather than one of the newer hybrid wheat varieties, and I could be confident that it wasn't genetically modified or plastered with pesticides. As with dairy, my pasta consumption went from "daily" to "rarely". I bought a rice cooker so I could cook the rice whenever I wanted, making it easier to have it readily available.

I incorporated oats, brown rice, wild rice, red rice, and the black "forbidden rice" into my diet. Plus complete-protein quinoa (seeds). Originally these were "acquired tastes" for me, but I did eventually acquire a taste for the nuanced flavors they offered. Soon, to my surprise, I actually started enjoying these grains more than pasta. My husband told me that "I told you so!" And yes, he did.

I have come to adore brown rice in particular, and I have a brown rice story:

*Years ago my husband used to come into the house each evening and ask "What is for dinner?" I liked pasta and he liked brown rice, but brown rice took so long to cook that my answer usually came back as "pasta". One night, he could take it no more and began shouting over and over again, "I want brown rice. I want brown rice!" I said, "Oh my God, it is only brown rice, why on earth do you like it so much?" to which he responded "Brown rice makes me happy!" I thought he was crazy, but following my nutrition studies I now know he's not nuts because brown rice makes me happy too by boosting serotonin production. How wonderful is that?*

## Gluten: Goodness or Glue?

Gluten is the prized protein that makes bread bounce. Well, it makes it *elastic*, which is why it found favor with bread makers and pastry chefs until it was deemed to be detrimental to health. Gluten is a complex and sticky protein that is difficult to digest for many people, and which is downright dangerous for those with celiac disease. Symptoms of gluten intolerance include digestive upsets, decreased energy, and an increase in cravings.

I feel much better when not eating gluten, and even switched to gluten-free oatmeal. Buyer beware: gluten-free fake food is still fake food, and I don't eat it.

## Switching from Sugar & Sweeteners

One of the big differences between my diet and the diets of my husband and children is that I used artificial sweeteners whereas they did not. I had used Equal for years, without realizing that it created havoc in my body. I learned that it was actually worse for me than the sugar it was replacing. It was a hard habit to kick, because the natural sweeteners recommended by Jeanette did not taste sweet enough to me. I did not know that artificial sweeteners register hundreds of times sweeter than natural sweeteners in the human body. It took some time to adjust to raw organic honey (the thick hard stuff) and maple syrup (grade B has the most minerals and flavor), but eventually these did become my staple sweeteners. I totally enjoy them and find their far more interesting and complex taste to be more satisfying and clearly more nutritious.

While I had never really been a sweet eater, I did indulge in the occasional cookie or cake. Oh, and chocolate. The sugar they contained became my "public enemy number one" insofar as how it immediately affected my body. I found I would go from happy at first, to sad within mere minutes (about ten of them). To stop feeling so unbalanced and unwell, I eliminated all candy and cake except for an occasional dark chocolate (preferably with nuts) plus an occasional holiday or birthday cake (to be sociable). Most importantly, I find that if I eat my sweet after a good wholesome meal filled with vegetables, the impact is nominal compared to eating that sweet on its own.

Sugar comes in several forms including glucose, sucrose, and fructose, which leads me to...

## Forgetting the Fruit

Despite being brought up on Grandpa Carmine's pomegranates, persimmons and other exotic fruits, even fruit did not agree with me. I found it hard to agree that it did not agree with me, because I loved fruit and ate a ton of it—including the habit, which my husband and I picked up from Grandpa Nick, of peeling peaches into wine.

I wanted to fit in with my family, and I wanted to honor those I loved so dearly by continuing their traditions and food selections. In this respect I knew that my internal resistance at least meant that I wasn't trying to change for the sake of change. But fructose (fruit sugar) was really not my friend, or at least no friend of my liver which had a great deal of difficulty digesting it.

I started to understand that my food needed to be chosen just for me, for my unique expression of a body. To quote magic wand seller Ollivander from the Harry Potter stories,

*"The wand chooses the wizard"* (rather than the wizard choosing the wand).

It was the same with food—more a case of which food likes me rather than which food I like.

So fruit went from *daily* to *rarely*. As dessert fare I occasionally enjoy nutritious organic and antioxidant blueberries, raspberries and strawberries. Plus I eat a few apples a week, a few figs, an occasional exotic mango or papaya, and some watermelon that contains mostly water (and very little sugar).

## A Whine about Wine

I love my wine but wine does not love me back. I *hate* that. One glass is okay; two is not. And every day is not okay. So I now drink a few glasses of wine a week, but I am still whining.

## Managing My Meat and Fish Intake

I was certain that my daily diet of fresh fish and pasture-raised meat was good for me, and I had spent many years finding sources of antibiotic-free lamb, venison, bison, beef, chicken, and turkey. Jeanette was convinced that I should nonetheless eat less of it.

I embarked on my next experiment—to assess the effect that meat was having on my metabolism. Once again, the results were very clear, but also very disappointing for the meat eater in me. I felt much more energetic, lighter, and I slept better if I refrained from eating meat of any kind. However, I satisfied my carnivorous cravings once a week with a very petite portion (2 to 4 ounces of any pasture raised or wild caught meat) combined with plenty of vegetables.

Having come from a family of meat-loving farmers and hunters, I thought that modifying my meat intake would be a modification too far. But it became easier and easier, and I enjoyed the fringe benefits of feeling less full and drinking less wine. My liver would surely thank me later.

On the other hand, eating fish made me feel fantastic, so I educated myself to eat only wild-caught fish including flounder, sole, salmon, squid, snow crabs, blue crabs, clams and cod... plus oysters, lobster and Gulf Shrimp. Our seas still offer a generous variety of healthy choices, and I enjoy seafood twice a week. But I rarely eat the same fish more than once a month because of the risk of repeated exposure to toxicity. I also reduced my sushi sessions from twice a week to once a month because it was raw and I could never be certain about the source.

## Better with Beans

As a child I did enjoy beans and lentils. I had been cooking them around once a week. I discovered, however, that my body enjoyed these far more often, and I began to eat beans or my favorite legume (lentils, especially the tiny black or green French lentils) at least once a day. As a fringe benefit, they are also easy on my food budget and offer affordable high quality protein.

My two favorite beans are black beans and chick peas, but I really do enjoy all beans.

## Happy Hen Eggs

I still remember collecting eggs straight from Grandma Rose's chickens, and Grandpa Nick would even drop a raw one in his beer. Fresh, organic, free-from-cages chicken's eggs without antibiotics provide happy protein. I always eat the whole egg because it is a whole food. I find this is a delightful way to encourage eating more vegetables, especially for breakfast. I cook up some onions, greens, mushrooms, and sauté an egg. I might put it all on top of some grains for a serious breakfast to fuel a big day.

Recent analyses demonstrate that these healthy eggs are not only more delicious, but also more nutritious. The healthy Omega 3 that fights inflammation is as much as 18 times greater compared to conventionally-raised eggs. I eat two or three a week.

## Seeds (and Nuts) of Change

For additional protein options I enjoy raw nuts (especially walnuts, pecans, almonds) plus pumpkin and sunflower seeds almost every day. I have also begun to eat chia seeds daily in my breakfast. The delicious complex flavors and extraordinary variety of different combinations make it easy to enjoy these nutrient-dense healthy food options. Some days I eat all of them in my quinoa or oatmeal!

I also have substituted grain- and nut-milks to replace all other milks (and no longer drink soy milk which does not actually agree with me).

## Vegetables: My Rock Star Food Friends

Jeanette suggested that half my plate should be green, plus salad on the side. Easy enough for me because I had grown up on my grandparents' greens, and I *immediately* felt the increased energy, clarity and improved digestion. I wanted to "go, go greens" more and more, and finally understood my husband's seemingly insatiable vegetable obsession. Yes, Cliff, you told me so!

I eat my greens with utter abandon—including dandelion, arugula, broccoli, broccoli rabe, avocado, escarole, frisee, watercress, chicory, kale, artichoke, bok choy, endive, green savoy cabbage, pea shoots, asparagus, and red tipped loose lettuce to name a few. I turn them into salads and soups, and often sauté them in garlic and olive oil.

I started to sense which foods were really healing me, and which were not. I noticed that truly whole foods – and preferably local foods – were my best friends. I referred to them as my *rock star friends*, because they were rocking my world.

Brown rice (wow!), quinoa, and oatmeal all make me feel fantastic enough, but I just can't count the ways in which I also love root vegetables. They ground me and nourish me in ways that I could not imagine any food could do. Quite literally, root vegetables keep me grounded, and I never tire of telling my friends and clients how important it is for them to have a good base of roots… just like a big strong oak tree. I love the depth of flavor and natural sweetness of root vegetables, with my favorites being beets, carrots, radishes, daikon, parsnips, turnips, and burdock. I would savor them in soups, or make a really good root roast. Just wash and roast the veggies, and don't cut them up until after they're cooked! Combine them with other "underground" foods including onions, sweet potatoes and yams.

The latest understanding of digestion is to understand and pay homage to our microbiome, our gut flora and fauna, which actually is in a symbiotic relationship with us and does the bulk of the digestive work for us. So, when I Increased my vegetable consumption (prebiotic) and especially fermented foods – probiotic like miso, sauerkraut, kimchi (note, from the refrigerated sections in the supermarket) – I increased the amount of happy bugs and decreased the amount of unfriendly ones. My grandparents dark dank garden dirt, I now understand, was filled with more than the creepy crawly bugs I delighted in seeing with my eye; also the zillions of health-promoting microscopic bugs that would make their way into our digestive tracts as a result of playing with the dirt and eating the vegetables grown on the dirt. This may be one of the best reasons for eating eat organic vegetables—not so much for the veggies themselves, but for all the friendly hitchhikers that conventional farming often destroys.

## Nightshade Vegetables and Inflammation

Macrobiotic practitioners refer to nightshades as "the deadly nightshades." It might be a bit exaggerated, but I know they increase inflammation in me and I believe they caused a problem for my grandparents who ate them in great quantities which probably exacerbated their arthritis. Pay careful attention to their effect on you. I only eat at most one serving a day, and skip them altogether if I sense any inflammation.

Nightshades include spinach, tomatoes, peppers, eggplant, zucchini, and white potatoes.

## Combating My Cravings

My body began to cooperate with me by starting to crave the cuisine that cured me. And conversely, by shunning the foods that failed me.

*Many years before embarking on my new food adventure, I had already learned to avoid cream. Some people said it couldn't be done, but cream made me so sick that I had started to see a metaphorical skull-and-crossbones every time I even thought about eating anything containing cream.*

The avoidance of cream set the scene for the more recent subtle shift in my eating habits. I stopped listening to my mouth and started listening to my body and its penchant for beautiful colorful and tasty food. I found myself in a condition of real connection with nourishment and nutrition, devoid of the deprivation associated with most "diets". What my food choices did have in common with alternative weight loss regimes is that *I began to lose weight*. Slowly at first, but surely I began to look and feel better.

I did not know I could feel this good. I began to feel vital and amazing. Great food, wondrously prepared opened me up to life and its celebration. I felt that every bite I took fed every cell in my body. Food that was energy-rich, vibrant and fresh began to make *me* feel energy-rich, vibrant and fresh.

*The "take away" message is that if you want to live your best energy-rich vibrant life, it is a great idea to take away (i.e. subtract) any food that is not nutrient dense and energy rich.*

## The Magic of Movement, and the Pursuit of Happiness

Think back to the beginning of this chapter, and you will remember that I hinted at the balance between energy in and energy out—between *food* and *movement*. So while feeling a little less fat, and already a little more fit, I set about satisfying my curiosity about the *magic of movement*. I had noticed a new yoga studio near my home, and decided to hit the mat. I also agreed to acupuncture with the extraordinary Dr. Gong from Beijing, and I resumed my work with the one-and-only Dr. Cliff Inkles—master maestro of the spinal cord and healing. These were monumental decisions, and you'll learn more about them in the next chapter.

To my utter delight, I had found that eating delicious joyous food (with a little walking thrown in) made me happy and healthy. Could *loving food that loved me back* really be the secret to a happy life? Could the pursuit of happiness provide me with the perspective and the philosophy that would form the cornerstone of my signature health coaching approach? This is, of course, a rhetorical question.

## 7 – Energy and Eastern Promise

In this east-meets-west chapter I tell the tale of how eastern alternatives to western medicine – along with a few new food friends – helped me defeat my demons and finally feel more worthy.

## The Power of Power Yoga

The work I was doing with Jeanette in 2012 inspired me to *move my body* by signing up at the 5Boro Power Yoga center located just a short walk from my home on Staten Island. My newly nourished (but still 200lb) body had been begging me to move it, but I thought I was too old and too fat to have a go. Intimidated as I was by the prospect of "power yoga", I signed up. To my delight, I discovered that I could do it. My yoga mat become my magic carpet; a safe place where my tears could combine with my dripping sweat.

Studio owner Karen Torrone (known simply as "Torrone") was a straight-talking tough cookie drill sergeant type, and very much the yang to her sister Susan's yin. Whereas Karen could break you down with a powerful program, Susan would build you up again with her gentleness and soothing essential oils.

Soon after I started at 5Boro, Karen ramped things up by offering a 40-day transformation program that was very purposefully designed to shake things up a bit. This program certainly did play its part in provoking change in me, and combined well with the work I was doing with health coach Jeanette. The new classes coincided with the loss of my best friend Jack, which heightened my sense of sheer emotion, so I welcomed the emotional support of the class participants even outside our classes. And I certainly needed that support, with so many emotions floating around in my body and around the room. I fretted that I couldn't cope with the physical and emotional pain of the program, and I even asked class co-leader Paulina,

*"Do you know what you're doing?"*

Then I remembered the mantra that would help me power through the power yoga program:

*Do the work!*

*Just do the work!*

## Essential Oil, and the Fruit Feast Challenge

The yoga class adopted a "group diet" that once more proved to me just how my husband was ahead of his time with his clean-for-decade diet. His only fear had been that, when preparing lighter food, I would deprive him of his *essential oil*—by which I mean his *organic cold pressed extra virgin olive oil*. How could this healthy thin man defiantly create "olive oil soup" at the dining room table? Once again he was in deep communication with his body, and completely right to ensure I did not remove this healthy fat from his food. It turns out that raw juice and salad diets don't contain the oils (avocado is a good one) that really are *essential* for absorbing the soluble vitamins in the vegetables.

Being part of my yoga group diet plan was fun but also posed an interesting dilemma. Part of this program was to do a group "3-day fruit feast", which left me torn between following the "integrity" of the program vs. listening to my own body. Not wanting to break from the pack of fellow yogis made me realize that this is the problem we all have, and the problem I had previously when following my grandparents' food habits: we all want to fit in with others, but sometimes we need the courage to also "fit out" by honoring our unique expression of our own body. So with some reluctance, I decided to stick with vegetables during the "fruit feast".

The more community-oriented yoga program was a nice interesting complement to the one-on-one counseling work I was doing with Jeanette. I enjoyed finding friends who were actively becoming *present* in their lives, and learning that they can create a more empowered future through intentional manifestations. My own manifestation was *this book*, which – I announced at our closing ceremony – would be titled…

**Fat, Fifty, and Fired!**

I'm glad I changed the title, as well as the emphasis on a much more motivational message.

## Adding In Acupuncture

Amazingly, right next door to the yoga center was Dr. Gong's Acupuncture Center. I crawled through the door practically begging for some relief from my intermittent anxiety. I found what I was looking for in the form of Dr. Gong and the healing techniques she had learned as a doctor in Beijing.

One day when I was getting my needles, an emotional wave welled up inside me. A tsunami of emotion. "Oh, I feel that," said Dr. Gong with amazing emotional empathy. My multitude of emotional traumas seemed to be being outed one-by-one by the yoga and the needles. These were the emotional traumas – from the terrorist attacks, hurricanes, and horrific battles with disease and pain – that I had previously repressed, and which I had merely bottled up to be let out later.

I went to yoga and acupuncture as often as I could go, since these seemed to be accelerating the energy and healing that I was getting from the food that was fuelling me. Although I was gradually feeling stronger, more powerful and even younger, I was seeking constant validation from other people.

*"Am I better?"*

*"Do I seem better to you?"*

When not asking questions, I was answering them, because Dr. Gong would ask for input.

*"Where does it hurt?"*

"Where doesn't it hurt?" I thought.

I helped her focus on my fatty liver and my ongoing war with worry and stress. The anxiety was so sneaky that it would disappear for days, only to reappear without warning. I called it my chest worm, because I could feel it starting to creep into my chest from my shoulders.

*"Oh my God, here it comes…"*

I felt the need to add some gentleness to my self-care protocol, and the yoga studio had the solution. Karen began offering a restorative class taught by Kira, which helped soothe and heal the body rather than activate and stimulate it. And the ever-gentle Susan with her big heart and *very essential* oils provided a serious infusion of comfort and soothing by offering slow movement and Yoga nidra (deep sleep) classes that placed me in a place of peace.

## Eastern Energy

These ancient Eastern modalities of healing are beyond wise. They are true gifts based on centuries of human wisdom, and they are directly connected to a deeper and truer understanding of our complex nature. They work on the premise that we are energy-based and that the energy can be directed.

Acupuncture assumes that the energy within your body runs along clearly defined energetic pathways that were identified thousands of years ago and recently confirmed with the advent of advanced technological imaging. The flow of energy can be altered by the insertion of needles anywhere along the Meridian pathway.

Yoga poses are also delightful in that they encourage us to grow by adopting a pose as a metaphor. Need courage? Do the "warrior pose". Need balance? Do the "tree".

We all know that *prevention is better than cure*, but we in the west often wait for serious symptoms to show up before we deal with disease. And this is exactly what I had done. But now I try to combine the ancient eastern healing modalities with my love of clean food fuel, to create balance and ease well in advance of any discomfort or disease. For those of us who sometimes need a break from "active" healthy healing, acupuncture allows us to just lay back and let the needles do their thing. Usually painless (with just an occasional pinch), acupuncture promotes a deep relaxed state as the parasympathetic nervous system takes over inducing a restful state which is when the healing abilities go into high gear.

In addition to acupuncture, Dr. Gong also administered the wondrous cupping—which is a real anxiety buster that I love. While it is also reputed to assist in detoxification, for me the best benefit is as a quick fix for anxiety. My wonderful reaction to cupping was intensified by an unexpected childhood memory of my Grandma gently pinching the flesh of our backs to help us fall back to sleep. So much so that I started to call Dr. Gong "Grandma Rose". The only downside was that the rubber cups which sucked up flesh like Grandma's hands left telltale red circles… which left my husband worried that people would think he was beating me up!

## Learning about the Foods that Loved Me Back

With more energy available to me, I was able to incorporate new cooking strategies and recipes that I really enjoyed and which connected to my heritage. I began truly to move in the direction of my embryonic "love food that loves you back" philosophy. I took pictures of my dishes, and started to share my recipes with others.

While I had to separate from some of the food that connected me to my family, their love of whole food provided plenty of possibilities for keeping the connection. Artichokes were a family passion and a must-have dish for every holiday. I became very articulate with artichokes:

stuffing them with quinoa and brown rice, steaming them, and using the leaves to dip in olive oil. I also used frozen artichoke hearts, canned artichoke bottoms, and jarred artichoke hearts in olive oil.

Amazingly I discovered that these delicious delicacies, regardless of how they were prepared, were amongst my favorite foods in the entire world… as well as the absolute healthiest supermarket selection, even when canned and jarred. It turns out that artichokes are from the magical thistle family, and are amongst the most liver-loving healing foods. My lonely liver – pining for its pal, my gallbladder – needed some TLC, so my artichoke intake went from *rarely* to *daily*.

\*\*\*

### Recipe for Artichoke Stew

Here is my recipe for artichoke stew:

- 1 bunch scallions (most potent antioxidant of onion family).
- 10 pearl onions (small white) peeled, stems trimmed, and left whole.
- 1 head of cauliflower florets.
- 10-12 whole baby carrots (or 4 medium carrots peeled and sliced into thin rounds).
- 1/2 cup olive oil, divided.
- 1/4 cup fresh lemon juice.
- 1 cup chicken or vegetable broth.
- 1/2 cup water.
- 10 artichoke hearts (substitute canned or frozen if needed) cut in half.
- 1/4 cup chopped fresh dill.
- Salt and pepper to taste.

Heat ¼ cup olive oil in a large Dutch oven over medium high heat. Add the scallions and sauté for about 5 minutes until tender. Add the pearl onions, carrots, and cauliflower, and continue to sauté the vegetables another 5 minutes.

Add the lemon juice, broth, water and remaining ¼ cup of oil.

Bring liquid to a boil, reduce heat and simmer covered for about 20 minutes or until the carrots are fork tender. Monitor the liquid levels and add a bit of water if needed.

Add the artichoke hearts and fresh dill and season with salt and freshly ground black pepper to taste. Cover and simmer for an additional 15 minutes or until the artichokes are tender.

Add sea salt and black pepper to taste.

***

I started to bring in other foods that my family and I loved. Only much more of them, and more often. I started to eat mushrooms and scallions every day, and lo and behold I made astonishing discoveries:

**Mushrooms** do not have to be eaten "occasionally" when foraged. Our supermarkets are filled with mushrooms, and I could even find the magic maitake mushrooms. As I learned more and more about my favorite foods to discover which were the healthiest, mushrooms came high up on the list, so I went from eating mushrooms weekly to daily. I even read how mushrooms have been implicated in protecting against cancer: particularly breast and prostate cancer, and particularly when combined with onions, which brings me to…

**Onions and garlic**, which are two more of the foods that definitely love me (and potentially you) back. I had often crushed garlic and let it sit in the salad bowl while I washed the salad greens, which I thought I did only for taste until I learned something amazing. When studying herbs with Holly Hayward of Sugar Hill Botanicals, I learned that this practice has a powerful practical purpose that was previously unbeknownst to me. When garlic is allowed to "activate" for 10 minutes or more, it forms a potent antibiotic called allicin, and four cloves of garlic are said to be as powerful as penicillin. Garlic is also antiviral, antifungal, anti-inflammatory and a potent antioxidant! Onions are equally amazing when it comes to their healing abilities as well as taste. The list of benefits from eating onions is long and impressive, and has been well known for centuries. I started to discover that cooking several onions as a single vegetable was totally delicious.

My other new vegetable friends included squash, escarole, sweet potatoes, beets, asparagus, and broccoli rabe. The latter comes with a story:

*Mrs. Esposito, my Uncle Fred's mother, was 83 when she told me this story. I had asked her the secret of her robust health. She told me, "I eat broccoli rabe every day, sometimes twice a day. I love broccoli rabe." She paused, then said "I guess it loves me!" Mrs. Esposito passed away just recently at age 103—some twenty years after telling this story, and after being sick for less than a year.*

***

### Recipe for Broccoli Rabe with Garlic and Red Hot Pepper

This is my favorite recipe:

- 1 brunch of broccoli rabe, roughly chopped with tough bottom stems removed.
- 3 tablespoons of unfiltered extra virgin olive oil.
- 2 cloves of crushed and chopped garlic.
- Dried red hot pepper to taste (I like it hot!).
- Sea salt.
- Fresh lemon to taste.

Quickly bathe the broccoli rape in boiling water for a minute, then drain. Heat a skillet on high and add the garlic and hot pepper, then add the olive oil and lower heat to medium. In a minute add the broccoli rape, some salt and a half cup of water or broth, stirring now and then for 5 minutes till tender. Squeeze lemon and enjoy warm or at room temperature.

OK—I cannot promise you that you will live to 103 like Mrs. Esposito, but I can promise that it is delicious!

***

## Losing Weight and Gaining Happiness

This was when I finally began to lose a lot of weight, sometimes as much as 1lb a day! I realized that my weight had been there to wrap me in a kind of emotional blanket, because my weight loss coincided with getting happy: a few hours here and there, and especially after eating a delicious whole food meal. My body, before, had simply not been willing to give up the weight and had been fighting me on every level.

The bottom line was that safety was a big issue for me, and I had to make my body feel "safe" after all the trials and tribulations that had affected my sense of safety. I learned that a human being cannot function at a high level without an internal sense of safety, and my poor *root chakra* (the root of my being) needed to be fully activated for my life to flourish.

## Essential Energy

Yoga and acupuncture propelled me into higher states of wellness. I decided to return to the *energy master*. It was time to return to Dr. Cliff, who had found the *path for life* for me (via Jeanette) and who my life's path had now led me back to. I had stopped seeing him when I believed I needed to first lose weight, so now, with my weight loss working out, it was the right time to return to my beloved teacher (and henceforth dear friend).

Trying to explain what Dr. Cliff does is difficult, because we are not trained to understand energy and its direct bearing on our being. At first I didn't understand how Cliff could ease the discomfort out of my body by barely touching me. But we are energy, pure and simple. We may seem solid, but we're composed mainly of open space and energy.

*I know what you're thinking—that this is pseudo-science bordering on bizarre mystic beliefs. But this is really real science. Look it up in any physics textbook, and you will find the "textbook answer" that the atoms which build our bodies are mainly empty space filled with energy that holds together the minute particles of matter.*

In an attempt to impress me, my dentist recently told me that "The future is energy medicine." I countered with the fact that energy and *energy healing* is not new; that energy medicine is thousands of years old, and that that many of the new energy healing modalities are merely rediscoveries. As a brilliant man in his own field of expertise, and with a clear curiosity, he didn't dismiss me out of hand... but didn't really have time to listen to everything I had to say about Dr. Cliff and his techniques.

Cliff is a trained chiropractor, but nothing he does – apart from treating your spinal column – reminds you of chiropractic work in the traditional sense. The founder of Network Spinal Analysis, Donny Epstein's work is so amazing that it seems it must have been channeled directly to him from another dimension. I am not expert on this work, but I am definitely a devoted patient.

*"As the spine and nervous system release chronic tension patterns, unlimited energetic resources come available to more readily assist healing and transformation in all aspects of life."*

Cliff and Donny are energy or "chi" masters. Their work takes you through stages of healing involving eliminating energy interference in your spinal column, *with no harsh manipulation*; merely movements, breathing exercises and gentle touching. Each stage offers a level of experiencing living that is associated with a pattern of thinking and an emotional state. I started in the sad state of being (moving in and out of suffering) that I had lived in for a long time, until I reached Stage 4 in which I was able to *get my power back*. The levels are not linear, up and down, but I felt a significant shift as I moved into what they called "advanced care": my feet became more firmly planted in reality, and I could actually see a new life stretching out in front of me.

I still struggled with worries about worthiness, and at one point Dr. Cliff assigned me homework to say "I am worthy" one hundred times. I learned so many lessons with Dr. Cliff, but this one was pivotal. Why am I telling you this? Because...

*If you want to change your life, you have to belief you are worth it, and I know you're worth it!*

I was rudderless; up the proverbial creek without a professional paddle. I love to work, but I did not know what kind of work was right for me in the shape I was currently in.

My prayers for work were answered by the ringing of my door bell. Saved by the bell, indeed, because it was my dear friend Ruth's brother, Philip, who offered me a position as a supervisor for his company. This would be the perfect position for me, since I would be helping hurricane victims. I was concerned about my lack of technical skills for the position, but I was determined to make it work.

Now the bad news…

## From Hired to Fired

I was still far too sick to work, and unfortunately this work forced me to figure out that I still had a long way to go to be well. I turned up, and tuned in as best I could, but I simply couldn't do the job. I found myself disorganized in this organizational role, plus technologically challenged, and totally stressed. The slightest slight from my boss would send the cortisol (stress hormone) coursing through my veins. With hindsight, I now know that my primitive *reptilian brain* – the amygdala – was taking charge by initiating my "fight or flight" response despite the fact that there was really nothing to fight or flee from. And my higher brain was consequently distracted from doing its job. This had been going on for years, but was masked by the maintenance of my brain's serotonin levels by the prescription pills.

The supervisor position only lasted three weeks but it felt like three years. I became discouraged, demoralized and demeaned. I also realized what an obsolete worker I had become when one of my staff, Lisa, on noticing that I didn't own a smartphone, looked at me with a mix of pity and curiosity as she said,

*"I have officially met a dinosaur."*

I had hitherto excelled as an executive in a world filled with helpful assistants who were experts with technology. I gave the first computer I purchased to my secretary, thinking of it as little more than a speedy typewriter. It was not that I did not think I could master the computer, I just thought it was not part of my job. Contrast this with the woman I had been in the 90's. My toy store in Florida was quick to develop a website, and I had done most of the work on it myself. That work had intrigued and challenged me, and I enjoyed the mind-numbing number of hours it took to learn how to develop a website. Now I did not even have a smartphone or a Facebook page. I had failed to learn new things and had fallen behind with the times.

Moving into the modern world would have been the logical thing to do, but – with all the stress hormones flooding through my body and my brain – thinking logically was not so easy for me.

Once I was fired (as kindly as my boss could manage) I knew I had a far more serious problem than I imagined. This was no small-scale temporary setback to bounce back from; this would require complete reinvention.

## The Road to Reinvention

Even though I had come so far, I was still really unwell, and I still needed external validation of how I was feeling inside:

*"I am getting better, No?"*

*"I am getting better, No?"*

My poor husband Cliff would try to console me:

*"Yes, Dorothy, you are getting better. You are getting much better."*

I was completely dependent upon the judgment of others. I could feel that I was *getting better*, but couldn't convince myself that I would ever *be better*... and *stay better*. While self-awareness is necessary for healing, I was more self-absorbed than self-aware, and disconnected from the real world.

I would faithfully go to Dr. Cliff and ask "What Stage of Healing am I in?" Then I would read and re-read the "Stages of Healing" book that described the mental and emotional conditions associated with the particular level. I felt better during my self-study sessions while working on transformation, and I realized that I wasn't transforming back into my old self... but into a *new me*. I also realized that the damage done to my body over decades could not be undone in a matter of days (or even weeks or months), so I needed to settle in for the long haul that would constitute the rest of my life. The problem of an *early death* had been replaced by the problem of living a *purposeful life*.

My nest was empty. My girls were now independent women pursuing challenging creative careers. Jessy moved from New York to LA and was busy creating a film career. Rose lived in Bushwick, Brooklyn and was a talented artist. I was proud of each of them, but missed them both so much. I longed for the little feet I used to pretend to take bites out of; their still-little feet now being frequently housed in black boots with no socks... and therefore far less appetizing than they used to be- still look awfully cute to me!

## The Institute of Integrative Nutrition

I wanted to go forward but did not know exactly where to go. What I did know is that I wanted to find a career that I could immerse myself in and become an expert, and which would allow me to make a difference to the lives of other people.

I prayed for inspiration (not for the first time), and it came in the form of the Institute of Integrative Nutrition: the largest nutrition school in the world, which offered the perfect program combining my love of healthy food with my desire to help others. I decided I would study nutrition with all of my heart, and learn how to dovetail it with other transformation techniques that would help me to holistically help other people. The program was online, and tests were conducted online, so students had to be relatively tech savvy. This "dinosaur" now needed a smartphone, an iPad and an understanding of social media. The first step to becoming an integrative nutrition health coach was to study radical self-care.

*I was still afraid and angry, and filled with regret. I knew there was something missing – a sense of happiness and joy that I experienced only fleetingly – but really had no idea how to heal beyond what I had already been doing. I could connect with Cliff (my husband) and my eldest daughter, but found it difficult dealing within anyone outside my inner circle.*

Studying brought great satisfaction. And while I continued in my quest to find an executive job, I carefully considered the real possibility of a "Plan B" purpose in life as a self-employed health coach. I didn't truly believe it (yet), but the mere possibility of this new purpose persuaded me to plow on with my studies. My otherwise lifeless life at the time was energized by the amazing lectures, the lovely energy of the students, and the zeal of the founder and faculty.

## Joining with Jeanette, and Training with Tom

As I began being kinder to myself, I found myself connecting better with others. My relationship with my health coach Jeanette grew in line with my growing confidence and knowledge base. I had such a sense of a renewed self that I remember sitting in her chair at one particular session, looking up, and seeing her as if for the first time. "Whoa, hello, it is so nice to meet you" I said as I shook her hand and she laughed. I wanted to study with Jeanette, to learn how to help others the way she had helped me, and I was delighted to move from *client* to *mentee* (with Jeanette as my mentor). I loved her "food first" perspective on healing, but also admired and understood how her program's "next steps" :

awareness and habit-shifting were critical for lasting change. I knew I had more to learn—for myself, and for my future clients. She could teach me that.

Jeanette did not have a formal training program, so she encouraged me to seek out the "next" level of healing arts by studying in the "Healer's Program" with Tom Monte—who was her mentor, and who she admired greatly. She knew Tom would accelerate my personal transformation, and prepare me to be a well-trained health counselor with a broad base of scientific information and a deeper understanding of ancient healing. In contrast with the Institute of Integrative Nutrition program that was online and could be studied whenever I wanted, Tom's program ran for six months and involved marathon study weekends in Manhattan. Could I possibly accomplish this? Or could I wind up making myself even more ill while trying to make the grade?

Within my small protected world I had begun to feel well. But outside my bubble, in Manhattan, it became apparent that I was far from well. Although I had lived in Manhattan for 20 years, I now felt confused and lost whenever I went there. The real issue, though, was that I felt a fraud by aiming for a level of academic performance and an associated new career that I had not actually earned.

## More Solace in Study

Whenever I felt unworthiness setting in, I would study as if my life depended on it. I truly found solace in study and became convinced that I should study as much as I could. When my brain wasn't busy, the worry set in. And when the worry set in, my body began to get sick. So to keep my mind (and by extension my body) healthy, I offered it what it wanted—information. I studied with Tom at weekends; I studied herbology with the knowledgeable Holly Hayward; I studied Reiki Japanese healing energy practice with JoAnna Crespo at the Open Center. I realized that a lifetime of challenging mental work would for part of my wellness protocol, and I continued to experiment with myself: food first, herbs next, add energy and study.

This new and growing body of expertise continued to make me a better, healthier human being as well as a better nutrition coach. As a better coach I began to feel worthy, and ready for more…

## 9 – From Slings and Arrows to Self-Love

People can tell us they love us, and this is wonderful. In the end, however, we really value the people who demonstrate their love not only by what they say but also by what they do. Lovingly feeding your body with health-promoting foods that you enjoy is a demonstration of your love for yourself. The *"Love Food that Loves You Back"* philosophy can also be used as a powerful practice to bolster and enhance self-compassion and love.

*It's no secret that self-love is a critical component for transformational healing, and it was a pivotal and difficult lesson for me to learn because I had worked so hard to care for those I loved or felt responsible for while clinging tightly to the life and position I was so attached to.*

## The Slings and Arrows of My Outrageous Fortune

Fighting and hanging tough had served me well in many situations. I thought surrender was for the weak, and that sheer hard work could solve any problem. After all, I had:

- Established a free senior citizen law clinic in Bushwick, Brooklyn at 24 years old.
- Founded a school in Battery Park City, lower Manhattan.
- Built two buildings and opened a retail store in Seaside, Florida.

By many people's standards I had been outrageously fortunate. But as every student of Shakespeare knows: *outrageous fortune* is usually accompanied by a barrage of life's *slings and arrows.* My own chaotic behavior compounded the chaos caused by the slings and arrows thrown at me during my decade of disease and disaster. And when the tide of my life turned, my talent for change deserted me.

I had been proud of being a "woman warrior" who could turn around any situation… *or die trying.* The only problem: *I was dying while trying.* And blaming myself.

The old approach no longer worked, so it was time to try something new. To learn a new kind of strength that was foreign to me. To replace self-judgment with surrender. To forgive myself, and to stop being my own worst enemy. To learn to love myself.

## Learning to Love Myself

My journey of self-love actually began in the doctor's office. His surprise message that I would not live out my life span had brought me in touch with emotions that I had previously either numbed or blindly vented when I could not contain them. I felt the fear, I felt the anger, and I felt the sadness. I felt the deep, deep feeling of sadness. Eventually, out of that sadness came the tenderness of self-love and compassion, and it was enough to get me moving—to get me searching.

Decades of emotions buried within my body began to release like demons… when doing yoga or getting acupuncture or working with Doctor Cliff. Little by little, though, these emotional releases brought me into deeper and deeper communication with myself.

I could feel the difference between self-blame (which was judgmental, harsh and cruel) and self-pity (which made me feel weak). I saw myself desperately wanting to replace the quick kneejerk reaction to blame others with the courageous act of taking responsibility to invoke a change in myself. The more I made these more enlightened choices, the easier it was to make them again.

I could also begin to better grasp and understand the language of emotions, and I began to engage these emotions not as enemies but as messengers to decode. As I developed an inner-world curiosity, I started to cut loose from my disabling anxiety. It seemed that putting just the tiniest bit of space between myself and my emotions, and asking simple questions like "What are you trying to tell me?", and truly listening, helped the messages flow freely. I realized I had caused myself a great amount of additional suffering simply because I did not give myself the time or the space to allow my emotions to express themselves.

Many women try to "hate" themselves healthy, and I realized that this was what I had tried to do too. I was so angry with the world and with myself. As I continued my journaling and my review of all the terrible things that had happened to me, I felt so much regret and shame. I thought to myself that I *should have done this… should not have done that.* My self-assessment was brutal and could make me sick for days on end. But Jeanette would guide me to a place of self-compassion for past "mistakes" that she referred to somewhat more compassionately as simply "missed takes"—things I would not have done if I had better understood the situation. It all made sense when I was with Jeanette, but within a few hours of our talk I would revert to self-hate.

As I became more self-aware, all my self-hate was uncovered, and it was startling. I had no idea about the magnitude of the big dark grudges I held against myself. Huge, angry, mean spirited grudges. I had taken it upon myself to be responsible for, ever since – at a young age – I had started to think that I was "in charge" of *everyone* and could fix *everything.* No one in my world was to suffer on my watch; everyone would be healthy and happy and would get everything they needed and wanted. It was perhaps no accident that I was once an advocate and attorney, since I would take huge personal risks to right other people's wrongs. Unfortunately, too many things had begun to go wrong. My subconscious belief that I was responsible for fixing everyone and everything had destroyed me and my life. I had no idea what toll it would take.

I started to understand the power that my subconscious beliefs had, and how important it was for me to know them and work with them. Then came the extraordinary and life shifting teachings of Tom Monte.

## Tom, Teacher of Teachers

Tom is a healer's healer, and was my teacher's teacher. Since he was mentor to my health coach Jeanette, I was already in awe of him even before I walked through the door, yet he still managed to exceed my expectations. Finding Tom was a huge blessing for me, and one which he would say was no accident. In (Tom) Monte's world, you are very challenged in life but also held in a state of love. You are safe in Tom's world as he ruthlessly works with you to bring your subconscious beliefs to the surface, and springboards your education so you can do this work with others. All the while, he holds you in a state of profound love and grace.

In Tom's classes we study relationships with ourselves and with others. He is an extraordinarily well-versed teacher. He combines the teachings of the latest science with ancient wisdom, and is able to deftly show how the two are weaved together into a tapestry that is well suited to healing people today. We pray and chant and get right to the "source"—whether this be God, Mother Nature, or your own particular higher authority.

Like all of my best teachers, Tom's teachings overlap and intersect with all the other lessons about life. In his class you start to understand that love is who we really are; and his promotion of love opens doorways into yourself that provide a pathway for compassion, forgiveness and growth.

But the cultivation of self-love can be elusive.

## Elusive Love

Like so many other people, I was engaged in a constant internal war with myself. When I really started to listen to the internal dialogue that plagued me – what Tom calls "the hungry thief" – I was appalled. When I heard myself internally saying "you fat slob" or "you idiot" I would think to myself:

*"Would you ever talk to a child of God like that?"*

As a child of God, why would I talk to myself like that?

So I sat down and started the process of loving myself by rewriting the internal script in my mind using the doorway of self-compassion. I could not believe the amazing effect it had on me, and I still cannot comprehend how a session of positive self-talk can instantly propel me into a state of wellbeing.

The key is to tell a version of the truth you believe. Self-delusions does not work... *although I had tried that as well.*

If I was tired or afraid, I would say to myself,

*"I love you so much. You are OK. You will rest soon. You are lovely and I am so proud of you for working so hard. It is okay to feel and fear, but you are profoundly loved and profoundly safe."*

Every time I heard myself being unkind to myself, I would change my internal dialogue to one of great compassion and love. It helped that I had a lot of experience of being a mother, so now I simply had to learn to mother myself.

The more I worked on loving myself, the more the quality and quantity of my love for others grew exponentially. It may be counter-intuitive, but it is true that the quality of your love for others is in direct relationship to the love you have for yourself. How could I possibly love my family any more than I already did? The answer was that it was not so much the quantity or quality of love as it was my own capacity. Love is an art and a practice that can only be expanded first within myself and then outside myself..

Tom worked with us on this. Tom exudes love, and with practice I could feel something really awesome growing within me—my heart was expanding and I felt walls coming down. And I began the critical exploration of my relationships with others…

## 10 – Loving Me, Loving You

Food continued to fuel me, but my relationships began to really fill me up. One of the joys of creating a banquet is to share it with the people you love.

## The Relevance of Relationships

We all know the importance of relationships with the pivotal people in our lives, and how these relationships affect our wellbeing. We also know the irony that the relationships most important to us are also often the most difficult. The people we love hold up the mirror of ourselves to us, and sometimes those reflections are what we do not want to see. I knew that my relationships with the pivotal people in my life had to be studied, and some had to be improved upon. With my own health returning, I wanted to "feed" the health of my relationships.

In my studies with Tom Monte, I was introduced to the study of traditional Chinese diagnosis of facial features. I was not too surprised to learn that diseases and body imbalances could be detected in a person's face. I was, however, surprised to learn how the health of a person's relationships could also be deduced from their face. In particular, the relationships with your parents are clearly evident. In my childhood I had sweet relationships with grandparents, parents, uncles, aunts and cousins. And then I had been blessed with a husband I cherished, and two girls who were my most treasured treasures.

*A favorite recollection of mine is of driving with Jessy in the car from Battery Park City to Staten Island when she was a toddler and I was still working on Staten Island as an attorney. On the way in one morning, I glimpsed the beautiful sight of her in the rear view mirror. Sitting in her car seat in the back seat, I observed that Jessy had a deeply dreamy expression on her face, complete with an angelic Mona Lisa smile with the sun gently kissing her face. It took my breath away. "Oh, honey" I said to her, "you look so happy and peaceful." She responded with "Oh,*

*Mommy. I am so happy Mommy; I am just looking out the window and seeing all of the pretty houses." I said "How wonderful... that makes ME so happy, too." She slightly furrowed her brow and got pensive. "No, Mommy," she said, "if you want to be happy, you have to look out the window and see the pretty houses yourself."*

My husband and I had a gifted life that we hadn't always appreciated. I always loved my husband and daughters, and Jessy's illness had given us a gift of treasuring each other and being gentle and kind to each other. But it had only lasted for short time before my husband and I began to grow distant from each other as the business problems became more and more serious. Then we lost EVERYTHING! Everything, that is, apart from what was most important—my beautiful, wonderful and very special family.

Relationships need to be tended with tenderness, and with tenderness comes healing. I realized that when I became sick, my relationships had gotten sick, so I decided to conduct a relationship review. In doing so, I found an amazing new source of strength to heal myself and my family. My relationships – like the people within them – needed to be big, loving, warm, healthy... and whole. I understood that these strong relationships would help us each weather our new storms.

## Reconnecting with Rose, and Winning the Unwinnable War with Cliff

In particular I had to mend my relationship with my younger daughter, Rose. We had gotten on odd terms with each other and had become distant. We quarreled all of the time. So I worked with Tom on this relationship, and something "clicked" when I revisited my motherhood. I got it. Rose needed a strong mother, and I needed to respect her for the amazingly young woman she was—to give her all the space she needed, and all of the unconditional love I had that I could give. Suddenly I could see how my communications with her had become one long whine, and how often the communication had been about me and my needs rather than her and her needs. I made the shift, and – just like that – the relationship changed. Tom said,

*"The love between you and your daughters is among the greatest gifts of life. Cherish it and each other."*

Gratitude.

Now I would have to turn my attention to the relationship with my beloved husband. Despite our differences, we had been a happy couple, but over time we had developed deeply held beliefs about each other that I knew were not true. We did not talk from our hearts very often, and we had been communicating with outdated *conceptions of each other* rather than to the *reality of each other*. But we did understand that we were changing, both were constantly changing, and that change was a good thing. One time, a friend said to Cliff,

*"Isn't difficult to be married to the same woman for over 30 years?"*

Cliff said,

*"What same woman? I have been married to at least eight different women, and who knows how many more women Dorothy will become!"*

In our early marriage we had "gotten" it for a while before the children were born. We were aware that we repeated the same arguments over and over again. We would joke:

*Why don't we just number the arguments so we don't have to waste our breath and energy repeating them? So the "toilet set cover raised up" argument could be argument number #3, so I would just call out "Number #3" when wanting to replay this particular spat.*

The silliness made us laugh.

But we shifted from those early, fun perceptions. Sometimes we cut too close to the bone when we traded metaphorical blows. I was terrified when out of work, and I was even more terrified that this time I would not recover. I wanted Cliff to *save me* and *protect me*, but I saw his flaws anew and started to deliver the kind of unkind and cruel prodding that only a loved one could deliver. I saw it, and was ashamed, but could not seem to help myself. I would apologize, but deep down I knew that I had to revisit this relationship in order to heal it. I wanted to *blame someone* for the problems I had created, and in particular I wanted to *blame him*.

I couldn't win this unwinnable war; I could only lose. Every hurtful blow I landed led to only humiliation and pain, and no pleasure at all. If Cliff stood up to fight me, I would stand by and be horrified by the damage I had caused to our relationship. If he simply stood by, calm and collected, I would feel embarrassed for my childish behavior. If I was "present" enough to see the absurdity of it all, it would change me for a time… until I was once again uncomfortable enough to lose my ability to be self-reflective.

## Seeing the Light… and Love

In my relationship studies with Tom Monte, I began to see new opportunities for awareness and growth. I realized to my horror that battles with my husband actually all began as battles with myself. I had to be willing to find the consciousness and presence to see what was happening before engaging in war with my partner. I began to see Cliff as he really was—my dear friend. We were both perfectly imperfect, and we would have to begin the process of falling in love again. I started to see his "flaws" as beautiful examples of his uniqueness. I started to see that I had choices. If an argument had started too quickly for me to process, I could still put down the sticks. If I knew I was uncomfortable, I could pause and make a choice. I began to see that I could choose between darkness and light. Yet too often I would still choose darkness over light, even knowing that there was no possible outcome that would please me in any way.

What was happening? How could I be wise enough to see everything, to know this much, but still engage in this self-defeating behavior? I realized there was a connection between my attempts to heal my relationship with food and my attempts to heal my relationship with my husband. It was willpower. I was trusting my most precious relationship to my elusive willpower; still relying on my small conscious brain to run the show. My conscious brain could indeed control my actions from time to time, but only until I became distracted or was under stress. Then my huge subconscious brain, aware that my conscious brain was no longer in charge, would start to pull my strings like a helpless marionette following some prewritten script that was entertaining no one. My subconscious brain was playing the preprogrammed response, Argument #3, and I wanted out of this program. But the more I tried to muscle out, the more entrenched my behavior became.

Then I remembered how I set about changing my relationship with my food. I started the internal exploration again. Feel what you feel. Discomfort. Anger. Fear. I could see that my preprogrammed knee-jerk reactions were based on fear. Seeing the damage my knee-jerk reactions were doing to me and other people brought me to a place of sadness… then self-compassion. Love. Light. Once I could let the light in, I could see more clearly and make better choices. THAT was the practice, and everything was connected to that practice. It was not about the food. It was not about the yoga. It was not even about the healing. It was all about love, and moving into the light. It was a grand dance, a beautiful ball, and I was invited. I felt humble and grateful and happy, and no longer a victim.

When my husband became cranky or angry, I tried to catch myself before I responded with negative emotions. Instead I tried to help him from my heart to find the cause of his dis-ease. In the gentle caring of him, I felt the strength returning to this pivotal relationship in my life. I felt so happy and so privileged, and I knew I would be well soon.

Then it hit me. We are nature. We do not merely *observe nature*, we *are of nature*. Like plants, we wither when it's dark. But we flourish when we are nourished, and we *open to the light… and the key is love.*

I had tried to live my life free from any practice that would acknowledge a connection with any spirit. For years I tried to create a life that was fuelled solely by my own mental muscle and willpower. I always had love for my family, but this didn't need any divine communion. I thought that asking for help from the divine was only for the needy and desperate. But that all changed with a little divine inspiration.

## Solace in Spirit

I now believe that just as we need to eat plants for our bodies to thrive, we are each by nature hardwired to bring the Source / God / Universe into our lives in order to achieve our fullest expression, and most importantly to feel the deep connection and unity that is the essential fuel for our soul. The potent powerful enlightening love is available and plentiful, and it is what we are born to grow toward.

Reconnecting to my own self-compassion led to the discovery of the food that nature intended for my body. Beyond that, it helped me understand the critical relationship between self-compassion, energy, and movement chi. The joy of health, which ignited and fortified me, moved me to better understand the critical nature of the relationships in my life. This self-love / food / chi relationship fuel was powerful and led me to a new career. *Something more* had called me.

Through my healing journey I came to the realization that I needed to reconnect to spirit in order to become fully healed. The love of "source" / "God" / "heaven", learning to relinquish "power", and learning to trust that I was  already profoundly safe and profoundly loved were necessary lessons for me to learn. That I was "in charge" had been an illusion, and that the effortful way I had conducted my life was only causing unnecessary pain and additional discomfort. The true test of courage was not in getting tougher, but in learning to *soften* and *open up* to the divine wisdom.

Opening up was not about giving up, but was about truly coming into a power that was the real source of all wisdom. We are just small drops of energetic love, and once we connect to our own love and that of others whom we love, the next step is to feel the enormous layer of love that envelops us. The "Little I", becomes the "huge everything".

I began to feel that everyone and everything is connected.

## Losing My Religion

I had lost my deep connection to spirit when I was a young girl in Catholic school. When I was around eight years old, my dearest friend Colleen and I decided to go on a mission. She had many dead Irish relatives, and she was quite concerned that many had been alcoholics and were probably languishing in purgatory in need of redemption. She decided she would save them. I thought she was so lucky because at the time all my relatives were alive, so she agreed we could share her abundant deceased relatives and she divided up their funeral cards for prayer.

During our school's playtime we began to sneak away from the Catholic school's grounds and would walk several blocks to our church. This walk in our suburban neighborhood on Staten Island was quite safe. The church was empty during this off-hour during the week, so we would sit down in a pew and begin fervent prayer:

*"Oh dearest Jesus, please free Mary O'Brien from purgatory."*

*"Oh Dear Blessed Mother, please, oh please, bring into heaven Michael Harris."*

And on and on, I would pray for Colleen's Irish relatives. We loved the good work we were doing, and we speculated on how many prayers might be needed for each of the lucky souls we were freeing.

Our work continued for a few weeks when, one day, the custodian of the church came bursting in, furious and yelling at us. He brought us back to the school. Other students came running over to us,

*"You are in trouble. You are in so much trouble."*

We were brought into the principal's office, surrounded by scowling and scolding nuns.

*"You know you are forbidden to leave the playground. We are calling your parents."*

Colleen was crying, but I was defiant. I kept telling them that we were praying. Praying really hard. Praying for all the souls that needed us. But the nuns were so focused on our safety that they neglected even to nod to our fervent mission. I remember feeling so betrayed that no one seemed to see the beauty or the importance of our project. I allowed that incident to rob me of the mystical communion that filled and nourished my spirit. Church lost its beauty as I began to suspect that those in charge really had no idea what they were doing. I thought that any communion with God would have to be a personal thing, and – other than an occasional joy-felt moment during a holiday mass – I lost interest in organized religion.

I did not give up praying, but the prayers became more of an internal form of comforting. I went through the motions during times of celebration such as weddings and baptisms, but without enthusiasm.

## Lost and Found (and Lost Again)

Having lost my love for organized religion, I began to reconnect to church and spirit as a young parent. When Jessy was first diagnosed with cystic fibrosis at the age of ten, we needed spiritual help. Although we got some advice and comfort from a therapist at the PS 234 Independence School in Tribeca, we needed more comfort. Jessy and I wanted to pray, and we wanted to pray in a church, so we joined the dark but impressive Trinity Church in lower Manhattan. Jessy and I loved Church. We felt communion and joy while sitting in the church during Sunday services. The spiritual energy would restore and heal our bodies as we sat together and held hands.

Cliff and Rose were heathens. Cliff preferred to sleep in Sundays, and attended only to support us (with evident displeasure). Rose, at the age of six, could only be persuaded to attend church by bribery: free hot tea after service, with me turning a blind eye to the 100 teaspoons of sugar she put in it. In contrast, Jessy and I attended for spiritual connection.

Our family stint as religious observants did not last long. The church had a lovely staff, our favorite being the warm loving Ms. Farina who was in charge of the children's religious instruction. The children's first event was to go to a movie about accepting gay friends. The church was also opposed to all wars, and I thought this was a perfect loving church for our aching family.

Unfortunately, a new vicar whom we dubbed the "vicar from hell" came to the church a year after our religious reconnection, and it served as a reminder that God's messengers could be a bit "off message". I was the president of the Battery Park City Parents' Association at the time, and had hoped that Trinity Church could find strategies to incorporate more member families from our neighborhood in Battery Park City. The Vicar was not interested in developing a community church or activities for the children. He was a lawyer and an accountant, and was far more interested in managing the assets of one of the richest churches in the world. He was dismissive and rude to other parents, and even to the lovely Farina who had presumed that – because he was a family man himself – he would take an interest in her children's programs. Everyone was upset with him, and he even started to respond to these issues from the pulpit on Sundays. Love and peace turned into politics, and we soon stopped attending.

Our family's religious experience once again turned non-existent. We thought that the girls had had a big enough dose of religion to understand the fundamentals of the Christian religion, and we thought it was enough now to be good loving parents. One Christmas morning, however, Rose asked why we celebrate Christmas. Cliff said that it was Jesus Christ's birthday, to which Rose responded by initiating the following conversation:

*"Who is Jesus Christ?"*

*"Jesus is the son of God."*

*"Who is God?"*

Feeling astonished that his younger daughter had no apparent knowledge of our religious and cultural background, Cliff went to a bookstore to find a children's book entitled "Who is God?" and started to read the book to the girls. Though concerned, I thought it was enough that we were raising lovely, caring, kind children.

Years later, after the disasters in Seaside, Florida my children did make me very proud and were the source of a huge testament to me and my husband; a testament that I will never forget and which was sorely needed when it was delivered. One of my angry creditors was loudly criticizing me in Modica Market when I happened to walk in. She immediately stormed out, and the lovely Mr. Modica rushed over to soothe me by waiting on me personally. I will never forget his kindness when he said to me

*"Dorothy, I have served many people for many decades and I have gotten to know a great many people. I have found that the best way to really know what a person is like is to observe their children. I know your children really well. And in my entire life I have never met finer children."*

## Guiding Lights and Missed Messages

My yoga practice brought the first renewed stirrings of religious or spiritual feelings within me. But it was not until my studies with Tom Monte that I began the critical work of reconnecting to love and following the thread to the source of our universe. Dr. Cliff's work also furthered my spiritual connection as the energetic blocks and emotional debris were cleared from my body. I learned the joy and pleasure of developing my spiritual connection, and it was again a pivotal lesson.

Now I fervently pray each and every day, much as when I was a little girl. I pray for family first, then friends, and then for the whole world. And I always remember not to "hang up" too quickly before *praying for me*. I am amazed how this communication with the *source of everything* comforts me and connects me with my "guides". Tom has also reconfirmed my innate sense as a child—that I have guides who love and protect me in this world. I now know that my guides helped me over the years, but I either ignored them or dismissed their help. One particular incident particularly demonstrated my guides at work:

*I had traveled to Seaside, Florida alone. It was the first time I had traveled alone for many years. Cliff, Jessy and Rose would be following me in a few days. I had to go sooner than them to have our house repaired from hurricane damage, and to get it ready for the upcoming rental season. I remember being exhausted; tired beyond belief. I walked into the house and did not even turn on the lights. I dropped my suitcase at the entrance and walked to the stairs that led to my bedroom. Turning left, and walking to the bookcase that was totally in the dark, I pulled out a book and tossed it into the garbage can. I continued up the stairs, took my clothes off and went to bed. I had no nightgown. I did not brush my teeth. I fell straight to sleep.*

*In the morning I woke to a beautiful, bright, sunny day. I went down and realized how odd it was that I did not turn lights on when I brought in my suitcase. Then I went into the kitchen to prepare coffee and breakfast. I saw the garbage can and felt a chill. I looked into the can and saw the small book I had tossed into it the previous evening. I picked the book out and started to read it. It was a book about a young teenage girl just a few years older than Jessy. This girl had cystic fibrosis just like Jessy, so no wonder I had been "guided" toward it, but why had I thrown the book in the bin? It turned out that the back cover told the tale of how this girl died at 15 (just two years older than Jessy at the time), so I put it straight back in the bin so that Jessy didn't discover it.*

Oddly I did not think about this again for many years, but I started to remember so many other missed messages and missed opportunities for connection, including…

## Dear Prudence

Albert Bruns, who had worked in my art store in Seaside, Florida was married to Prudence Farrow Bruns. Prudence was the subject of the Beatles song "Dear Prudence." During one of the hurricane disasters in the summer of 2005, Albert had reached out to me for a favor. He asked if his family could stay in my Seaside home during one of the more powerful hurricanes of the season. Our house was made of concrete, and he felt his family would be safer there. I was happy to help, and they were grateful. In a kind gesture, Prudence offered to teach me transcendental meditation. The truth is—I was always uncomfortable with people who had any fame. I simply felt shy with Prudence, and sincerely felt I had no time to learn mediation and had no time to practice. Ironically, I thought I was far too "far out" (stressed and crazy) to have time to learn meditation.

I was on my yoga mat at 5 Boro Yoga when I thought about Prudence's offer. I did not learn meditation back then, but why not try to reach out to Prudence to learn now? Mediation was resurging in popularity, I had read many positive reviews of Transcendental Meditation (TM), and one of my prayer cohorts from my healers' group was a fervent believer of the benefits of TM. I looked up Albert on Facebook and friended him, so that (by extension) I could send my own "Dear Prudence…" message to dear Prudence and straight-out ask if her decade-old offer still stood.

At my next yoga class, instructor Kira (to my surprise) was playing the song "Dear Prudence". I first thought I must have told Kira about my idea to contact Prudence, but I realized that no one had known about me reaching out to Prudence only an hour before. Kira looked clueless when I asked her how she knew to play this particular song.

*"Dorothy, I have no idea what you are talking about, and this is probably only the second time I have ever played the song Dear Prudence in yoga class."*

Just a happy coincidence, then. Or maybe something big showing up, because when I got home there was a message from Prudence. She told me that, although her TM course fee could not be waived, she would love to teach me transcendental meditation, and would be happy to fly into New York City to train me.

## Transcendence

The storms started as soon as the night came for Prudence and Albert to arrive. The late night flight came in deep into the early morning. The airport was flooded, and I felt flooded with cortisol (the stress hormone). I wondered if I had made a mistake, but as soon as I saw Albert and Prudence I felt relief and even joy. Prudence was wearing her jeans, cowboy boots, and a warm welcoming smile. She had a lovely peaceful manner and I knew instantly that the trip was going to be perfect. I could not be happier to see my old friend Albert, who used to do transcendental meditation on the roof of our building, and it filled me with joy to remember the fun days at Quincy's. He recounted how insane it was to work there—with Jim demonstrating the wind-up tin toy duck, kids covered in paint from one of Lloyd Ann or Lisa's art classes, and Arix and Tom demonstrating Mystix Juggling Stix. Our "Please touch, please play, and please have fun" attitude was a bit madcap, but I had loved it and loved being reminded of it. Our customers loved it too, and I remember a young boy one day coming into the store for the very first time. He walked in and spun around, eyes wide open, swallowing in the unusual offerings: the marionettes designed by artists, bright colorful art supplies, Japanese kites, tin toy collections, scooters, juggling gear… and so much more. He raised his arms to the heavens and shrieked "I have died and gone to heaven!"

*The business venture had made me very happy, but never made me much money.*

I had no idea what the TM induction ceremony would be like. It was quite magical, wonderful, conducted in Sanskrit and involving flowers and fire. The students arrived one-by-one, all on time, and we worked from 10am to 11pm. Prudence was perfect as the "real deal" expert. I was thrilled to get my mantra and start my practice, and the wondrous part was that the practice was not difficult at all. But it was subtle, such that training with an experienced teacher was imperative. We all learned to our delight that Prudence was the longest-trained teacher, and had been trained herself (of course) by the Maharishi.

For three days we all met at Dr. Cliff's, and time seemed to be suspended. When all was over we were so sad to see Prudence and Albert go. We all hoped we would see each other again, and it may yet happen, but the magic of the meditation was already starting to set in. My brain began to work well again. I seemed to be able to organize, plan and execute plans in a more effective manner. I began to have clearer focus and things began showing up for me. I acquired new clients, new relationships, and was afforded new opportunities.

I can say that ever since I began meditating and fervently praying, amazing things have happened:

- I opened an integrative nutrition health coaching practice in New York City.
- I offer health coaching to people around the world via telephone, Skype, and via webinars.
- I am a featured speaker at wellness retreats, organic farms, businesses, and organizations.
- I am teaching classes on nutrition, self-health, and writing.

I discovered that when I opened to my guides and softened my heart, life began to show up differently and transformation kicked into a higher gear. I am not only healing, but also thriving.

## Gift of Guides

Earlier in this chapter I alluded to the gift of guides that have lovingly guided me and continue to do so. The more mindful I have become, the more I have remembered and reconsidered my guides' communications with me. These communications had several shared attributes:

- They always seemed to come out of nowhere.
- They were not part of an actual conversation.
- They seemed separate and distinct and sudden.
- They were kind, and often funny, but always enlightening.
- They were unusual and always perfectly timed.

I have already shared some of my guides' gifts throughout this book, and here is a recap of those communications:

*"I love mimosa trees but I love you more." (Grandpa Nick)*

*"I love broccoli rabe, and it loves me back." (Mrs. E)*

*"Look out the window yourself, Mommy." (Jessy, looking out of my car window)*

*"Hate makes more hate." (Jessy and Rose, days after 9/11)*

*"Brown rice makes me happy." (Cliff)*

*"Judge people by their children; you have the finest children." (Mr. Modica)*

The guides' helpful communications did not necessarily come in the form of quotes. Sometimes they came in the form of happy coincidences:

*The Cystic fibrosis book in the garbage.*

*The bus driver who prayed for my cats on my behalf.*

*The yoga studio just down the block.*

*Teacher Tom Monte.*

*Prudence offering to train me in transcendental meditation.*

*Dr. Cliff handing me the "Path for Life" card.*

*Jeanette and Dr. Gong offering for me to use their offices to start my business.*

There were so many more; hundreds more. I have been surrounded by loving teachers and guides my entire life, I just did not see or understand. I do not know the *how*, *why*, or *who* of these communications, and my logical mind is mystified by them, so I have learned to ignore my mind and follow my heart.

I remember one more: the way my doctor's physician assistant Keith blurted out,

*"You are not going to live out your lifespan."*

It had that same mystical magical quality.

## 12 – The Doctor, the Diet, and the Secret of My Success

Over the past several years I had visited my doctor's office regularly. Past visits had been painful, so it was such a wonderful surprise when my efforts were rewarded with the following words:

*"You are a miracle. You are a new human being."*

Each new visit brought another new wonderful surprise.

One-by-one I was taken off of all of my medications. Pound-by-pound I was losing weight and getting thinner. Every visit I was healthier, and each time I felt better. Most importantly, my life was clearly becoming fully nourished.

It was clear to me that by "loving food that loved me back" I had changed my relationships to myself, to my food, and to all other aspects of my life.

Keith (the doctor's assistant) was eternally elated, and even in awe.

*"You are on no medication. You lost over 70 lbs. And you blood work is nothing less than astonishing: glucose levels steady at 80, and triglycerides down from 230 to 120.*

*You do not understand. This does not happen. Ever! It is like you created new human being. You are a miracle.*

*You did this by eating plants? By simply eating more vegetables? And you love this food? Really Dorothy, really?!*

*What happened to your depression? What happened to your anxiety? Is it really gone? Are you really feeling that good?"*

I told him the truth:

*"I have a bad hour or two, but I know what to do to bring myself back in balance. I usually only have to eat some delicious food, maybe do some yoga or take a walk, to get back into balance.*

He looked over at me.

*"How much do you charge? I am going crazy with so much stress. I know I should eat better and take better care of myself. But I am so busy, I do not know where to start."*

I did not understand what he was saying to me. Then he gave me his email address, and suddenly I got it. Keith was considering hiring me. ME! I was excited and delighted, but then I looked at him and felt his pain. I remembered feeling that pain.

*"Please believe me, Keith, it really is all true. Food matters. Food is foundational for health. Vegetables are the key—there is life in them, there is medicine in them, and we were born to eat them. Plant cells and human cells evolved together in a symbiotic relationship. We take in the oxygen that trees (and other plants) create. Trees take in the carbon dioxide that we breathe out.*

*Our complex bodies are designed to need the many parts of plants: the phytonutrients that heal us, and the fiber makes us thrive. And the very best part is that plants are delicious as well as delectable. The more you eat them, the more you want to feel their magic. Oh, Keith, I really wish I had started a lot sooner. I still mourn my missing gallbladder, but I am grateful to have finally 'got there' and I am so grateful to you... my friend.*

*I know all about it Keith. It is so hard when you are so busy, and the hardest part is to start. But once I reached out for help, the help was at hand in the form of my kind coaches and teachers. I would honored and love to help you."*

And dear readers, I would be honored and would love to help you too....

## The Secrets of my Success

*Note that this is what works for me, but it might not be exactly what works for you. It's a good general guide, but everyone is unique, and you need to discover you own blueprint for good health.*

## Drink Do's and Don'ts

I drink a lot. Not so much wine these days (whine!), but I drink plenty of clean filtered or spring water… ideally not out of thin plastic bottles that leach hormone-disrupting chemicals. I shoot for drinking about ten eight-ounce glasses a day. Most of us are dehydrated, creating body havoc, even stressing our internal organs, and which is why I fill myself with fluid.

*To test for dehydration, pinch the skin on the back of your hand—if it doesn't snap back, you might be due a drink of water.*

As well as the Plain Jane water, I drink:

- Green tea, which acts as both an antioxidant and an anti-inflammatory. The tiny caffeine kick is nowhere near as concentrated as coffee (which is anxiety-in-a-cup for me). After 4pm I only drink herbal tea, which counts towards my water content.
- Fresh vegetable juice or a smoothie a few times a week, which would be more if I did not already fill myself with 8-10 vegetable servings per day (with fresh avocado or olive oil to help absorb the fat-soluble vitamins).
- Water with lemon, to start the day and help detox my liver. Other "spa" additions include lime, mint or cucumber.
- Nut milk or grain milk from time to time, and often on oatmeal or cereal, but avoiding the potentially cancer-causing carrageenan additive.
- A few glasses of wine per week, and an occasional dark beer (with food to dampen the effect of sugar on my system). *Wine tip—start to*

*add water when the glass gets half empty, to create a pretty blush drink to finish up the meal.*

I don't drink:

- Commercial fruit juice or soda, because of the sugar content.
- Coffee, except as a rare treat, and especially not for energy which is better obtained by getting in my greens.

Looking to lose weight? Then you might be interested to know that I sometimes tended to eat when I simply felt thirsty. So next time you're hungry, reach for the refreshing water first to quench your thirst.

## Food Facts

Okay, so you can't fill yourself with fluids alone. Here I present the facts about the food I eat, starting with *when I eat them.*

### Timing

I eat three meals a day at specific times: 7am-8am for breakfast, 1pm-2pm for lunch, and 7pm-8pm for dinner. I would actually like to eat dinner earlier, but I prefer to eat with my husband when he comes home for work. It is important for me not to deviate, so I prioritize and plan for this. I eat enough at each meal to keep me nice and full until the next meal time.

Why? I think it is easier to know and plan what you are eating at a designated meal time. My body has learned to count on me to feed it, and to feed it nutrient-dense and delicious food. I have developed an internal rhythm that is comforting and which establishes a deep sense of security. When I grazed, it often resulted in eating too much or not enough (and erratically) thereby increasing my anxiety and unbalancing my metabolism.

Most of what I eat is a habit, but with three or four choices built in for variety. *Breakfast-Lunch-Dinner* is my concept of laying down food habits to support you, so that when you are distracted you can go on "autopilot" knowing you will be fed well. I enjoy every one of my meals and can depend upon feeling great after I eat them.

## Enjoyment

Enjoyment is an important component of *loving food that loves you back*! Not only do pleasure signals help with healthy habit-forming, but also studies have shown that *enjoyed* food may be absorbed 40% more effectively. "Yuck" signals our cells to beware, whereas "yummy" opens them up to enjoy.

## Reversing the Concept of Contorni

Earlier in this book I told you how in Italy vegetables were called "I contorni" because they were intended to contour or round-off a meal. Indeed, in my early life I regarded protein (meat / fish) or refined starch (pasta) or rice to be the main component of any meal. Now I have reversed this concept such that if you ate at my restaurant (I don't have one, yet) you would order a *main course of vegetables* with *small side dishes of protein and whole grains.*

## The Meals

Enough about the generalities of my eating habits. Now what about those meals?

My **breakfast** comprises most of the whole grains that I consume each day—usually oatmeal, but sometimes brown rice or quinoa (a complete protein source, and actually a seed rather than a grain). I add a nice variety of seeds and nuts: pumpkin seeds, sunflower seeds, walnuts (high in Omega 3), almonds and chia seeds (also a super food and high in Omega 3). My Sunday breakfast is usually a big vegetable sauté and a nice farm fresh egg with some brown rice. I may go mad at the weekend... and have a nice organic sourdough, wholegrain piece of toast.

I never ever skip breakfast, because – if I do – I eat all night!

For both **lunch** and **dinner** I eat vegetables in earnest, and I always think first about what vegetables I want.

I include at least one of either vegetable soup or hearty vegetable salad, and by "hearty" I mean not merely a few leaves of iceberg combined with cucumber and tomato. The salad has to have at least two or three green or red leaves – prewashed in the refrigerator – and my favorites are watercress, kale, arugula, red tipped loose lettuce (a surprising powerhouse of phytonutrients even though it is nice and soft), dandelions, spinach, endive, radicchio, romaine, cabbage. Then I add the "goodies" including olives, artichoke hearts, carrots (some raw, some cooked), beets, cabbage, Brussels sprouts (can shred raw or steam), asparagus, cooked mushrooms, steamed broccoli or cauliflower, or leftover squash.

I often add root vegetables, onions, squashes and I always eat plenty of garlic—which I activate by chopping and letting rest prior to cooking. I eat mainly *sweet* potatoes rather than white ones, but I learned a fun fact about white potatoes. When chilled, these potatoes convert the sugar that is ordinarily released quickly into your system (thereby creating a high glycemic situation) into a form not readily absorbed. So now I always cook and chill white potatoes, and eat occasionally in a nice potato salad.

I eat plenty of beans and lentils, and I add some fish a few times a week. I also add whole grains. While whole grains make me happy (I love brown rice!), I eat less of these than vegetables. Half a cup is just fine.

I eat some probiotic food each day, either some miso soup, sauerkraut that I add to salads, or one of my favorites—kimchi (hot and spicy).

Sweet and Fat

No, I'm not referring to the old me!

When it comes to sweeteners, I never use artificial ones. I use grade B real maple syrup and raw organic honey. Dried fruit (especially the delicious majool dates, apricots or cranberries) can be fun to add if you need some sweetness.

We need fat, and the right fat (not trans-fat) makes you healthy… not fat! I love olive oil, and use it 99 percent of the time for our fat requirement. I have found that the less processed unrefined extra virgin olive oil, which is starting to become available, does not smoke as readily. Another trick I use to reduce the chance of "smoking" (creating toxic chemicals you do not want to consume) is to heat the pan first, then add veggies or whatever else you are cooking, and then reduce the heat before you add the olive oil. Another trick is to add fluid (vegetable or mushroom broth) first after heating the pan, and then drizzle on some olive oil after the cooking. I also like untoasted sesame oil and avocado oil, and in fact I eat whole avocado (not just the oil) frequently. My skin and brain both thank me for the fat.

## Keeping It Real

I mean this in two senses…

- In the first sense, I do my very best mostly to eat *real* whole food in natural shapes; e.g. carrots that actually look like carrots. I also do my very best to eat local organic food, which is best for our bodies and preferable for the planet.
- In the second sense, I mean "keeping it real" by not getting obsessive about this. If you can't find or afford organic fare, then non-organic vegetables are still far better than anything you will find in any processed "convenience" cuisine.

The best clean nonorganic vegetables to eat are as follows: asparagus, avocado, cabbage, cantaloupe, cauliflower, eggplant (nightshade), grapefruit, kiwi, mangoes, onions, pineapple, sweet corn, frozen sweet peas, and sweet potatoes.

The dirty dozen (most polluted) vegetables that you should make every attempt to buy organic are as follows: apples, celery, cherry tomatoes, cucumbers, grapes, nectarines, peaches, potatoes, snap peas, spinach (nightshade), strawberries, sweet bell peppers (nightshade), hot peppers (nightshade), kale and collard greens.

Still on the subject of keeping it real, I admit that *I am not perfect.* I eat 90% healthy whole food and I love it. I avoid becoming too rigid, and on holidays and birthdays I do indulge in a celebratory slice of cake or a cookie. If I am cooking the treats myself, I make them with healthy organic ingredients and healthier sweeteners. And I do eat some dark chocolate from time to time, which really take the time to savor.

## Movement and Meditation Magic

As indicated throughout this book, it's not only about the food. I have also discovered the magic of movement and meditation.

### The Magic of Movement

I get off my bootie as often as I can, and I do not let my body energy stay stagnant. I try to build in bursts of energy: madly dancing around (not in public) or jumping on a trampoline a few times a day. I do my power yoga three times a week, and the more active I am, the easier it is for me to keep anxiety and depression away.

Activity doesn't have to be quite so active, and movement can be a little more modest. I enjoy a bi-weekly walk in nature. I love my restoration yoga, and yoga nidra at my yoga studio with my yoga community. If I cannot get to the studio, I practice on my yoga mat at home.

If I feel any dis-ease (as in feeling uneasy) within my body, and if exercise has not done the trick of dislodging the "stuck" feeling, I go to Dr. Gong for acupuncture or to Dr. Cliff for spinal release. I usually visit either or both of them twice a month, but the better care I take of myself, the less often I feel dis-eased (as well as diseased) in the first place.

Acupuncture, spinal release, and even yoga take us from the *magic of movement* to…

## The Magic of Meditation, Tapping into EFT, and Talking in Tongues

I experience the magic of meditation twice a day; becoming clear and counting on my consciousness. The more I become aware of my true needs, the more I am "present" to take good care of myself, my family, my friends and my clients. Everyone benefits when I show up loving and happy and whole. Meditation and prayer combine well together, and each day I pray for myself, my loved ones… and the world.

I also study, I enjoy practicing Reiki, and I have learned to "tap" into the power of the Emotional Freedom Technique (EFT, also known as "Tapping"). EFT facilitates communication with your subconscious, which helps you drive your life forward without being hijacked by the huge subconscious and highly programmed brain that thinks it is keeping you safe when really it is keeping you trapped in predictable patterns of behavior.

I am not afraid to experiment with anything that may be helpful and health-full on my life's journey. At a recent meditation session I was encouraged to fervently talk in tongues for fifteen minutes before bed, to deprogram my subconscious for a better night's sleep. Quite loudly I went from Italian to Chinese (or something like it) to something much more animalistic. Cliff slid into bed beside me and began reading. I said,

*"Oh, I'm sorry Cliff—that must have been so disturbing for you."*

With typical understatement, he responded,

*"Honestly, Dorothy, it wasn't that different from your usual conversation"*

I hugged him and bellowed out a belly laugh, because I hoped he was just joking!

Jokes aside, laughing is good because it releases happy healing hormones called endorphins that make you *feel good about yourself.* And hugging is healthy because it releases the "love" hormone oxytocin, which makes you *feel good about other people* and your relationships with them. Oxytocin also opposes the stress hormone cortisol.

## My Health Heads-Up

Once again, I mean this in more than one sense. I wanted to conclude by giving you a "heads-up" on my health today, but I can confidently say also that my health constantly "heads up."

Today I am so blessed. My health has not merely returned, but has exceeded anything I ever knew before. I take great pleasure in continuing to tinker with how I take care of myself—which has become a journey rather than a destination.

Our mind, body and spirit, and their interconnections with the intricacies of life are truly amazing. For many years, this beautiful but abused biological miracle of my body worked so hard to take good care of me while I ignored and neglected it. Now that I am conscious, I am committed to rectifying this wrong and have developed a reciprocal and loving relationship with my entire self.

So what is the secret of my success, which has led to a state of exponential healing?

*The simple secret of life is to be found in life. In nature. Be in nature, understand nature, and understand that you are nature. Eat things that grow, and then grow yourself.*

*Love food that loves you back, because life fully nourished is delicious.*

\*\*\*\*

Come visit my website at www.nurturenaturenutrition.com for free offers or to contact me. I am offering new delicious recipes and nutrition tips. I am also offering private and group nutrition and nourishment counseling, plus original and fantastic retreat and class opportunities. See you there!

Or contact me at coachdorothyholtermann@gmail.com.

Because life fully nourished is delicious...